1,0(

FOR THE PARENTS OF

AUTISTIC

BOYS

1,001 Tips

FOR THE PARENTS OF

AUTISTIC

BOYS

Everything You Need to Know About Diagnosis, Doctors, Schools,
Taxes, Vacations, Babysitters, Treatment, Food, and More

Ken Siri

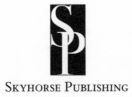

SKYHORSE PUBLISHING

Skyhorse Publishing books may be purchased in bulk at special discounts for sales promotion, corporate gifts, fund-raising, or educational purposes. Special editions can also be created to specifications. For details, contact the Special Sales Department, Skyhorse Publishing, 307 West 36th Street, 11th Floor, New York, NY 10018 or info@skyhorsepublishing.com.

www.skyhorsepublishing.com

10 9 8 7 6 5 4 3 2 1

Library of Congress Cataloging-in-Publication Data

Siri, Ken.
 1,001 tips for the parents of autistic boys : everything you need to know about diagnosis, doctors, schools, taxes, vacations, babysitters, treatment, food, and more / Ken Siri.
  p. cm.
 ISBN 978-1-61608-105-8 (pbk. : alk. paper)
 1. Autistic children. 2. Boys. 3. Child rearing. 4. Parenting. I. Title. II. Title: One thousand one tips for the parents of autistic boys.
 RJ506.A9S568 2010
 618.92'85882--dc22
         2010038845

Printed in the United States of America

For my mother and father who made all possible,

and

for all the parents out there fighting to improve the lives of their kids.

Contents

Contents

Introduction

I wrote this book for two reasons: first, to educate myself on how best to organize the challenging life of a single dad of an autistic boy, and second, to share what I've learned and provide a shortcut for those who follow.

You will notice that the section headings utilize both clinical and combat-laden terminology which I've borrowed from Sun Tzu's *The Art of War*. Parents of autistic children need to adopt these mentalities. While you must become analytical like a clinician or scientific researcher, you must also become a warrior, fighting as if you were a soldier on the front lines, because in many ways, you are.

This book confirms that there are many services and organizations available to help you, but you will learn that, in the end, you are both general and soldier in this fight. You must take ownership of all aspects of treatment, education, therapy, and organization as if preparing your army for battle, and you must also fight in the trenches for your child, because if you don't, nobody else will. The "squeaky wheel gets the grease" may not be fair, but that is the way you must fight this battle with autism, so be ready for it.

Besides having to fight like a warrior for your child, you will also experience the stress that accompanies the battle. A recent study revealed that when parents of children with autism were stress-tested and compared to various professional occupations, the closest equivalent they could find was that of combat soldier. Not just a soldier, mind you, but one in combat. Basically, we are under fire, 24/7. This book will discuss how to fight, but also, how to handle the accompanying stress; how to manage the services you will seek; and how to deal with a society that remains, despite ever-increasing awareness of autism, largely ignorant of what our lives are like.

Battling autism can leave one feeling devastated and alone. You will need help and support along the way. Many parents are going through what you are feeling and dealing with right now. I hope that this book will educate, aid, and, most important, remind you that you are not alone, and that there is hope out there. Let us begin!

Author's Note

This book seeks to provide helpful tips, general information, and strategies to help families master autism. This book is not intended to provide specific medical advice; all therapies and treatments discussed are for informational purposes only. If anything in this book conflicts with your doctor's advice, you should follow your doctor's advice. All medical treatments have the potential for harmful side effects, so seek the advice of your doctor before beginning any biomedical treatments for your child.

Autism is a spectrum, and all children with autism are different. What works for one child may not work for another. For this reason, some of these tips may appear to be contradictory. As a parent, your first job is to get to know your child, and in doing so, you will have a better idea of which tips in this book will apply to your son.

These tips have come from various sources, and we have kept the voice of the different contributors. In doing so, we realize that different terminology is used when describing children with autism (autistic child, child with autism, child on the spectrum, aspie, child with Asperger's, high-functioning, more-able, more-impacted, etc.). Just remember: A rose by any other name smells just as sweet . . .

These are tips and not rules, so try them out and adopt what works best for you and your child.

Note that the book is organized by autism chronology, so that those beyond the early stages of diagnosis can skip to the tips they need. Tips are also numbered for the sake of reference.

1,001 Tips

FOR THE PARENTS OF

AUTISTIC

BOYS

....

Pre-Diagnosis—Strategic Assessment

Our first set of tips focuses on early signs and symptoms of a possible autism spectrum disorder (ASD). Consider them your scouts and an early warning system.

CHAPTER 1
Early Symptoms of Autism Spectrum Disorders (ASD)

1. If you have any inkling that your child's development is off, it should be handled at the youngest possible age, as we now know that early intervention leads to better outcomes. Bring to your pediatrician's attention any apparent delay or symptom (see list below), and do not accept "It's a phase" or "Don't worry" from anyone. Seek a second opinion if necessary!

2. There are many lists out there describing symptoms of autism, feel free to Google for more. We present a sample grouping below. Review, and if you note any delays see your pediatrician. Remember to err on the side of caution; it will help you catch any issues early when prognosis is better.

Speech Problems:
- Nonverbal (unable to speak, perhaps has a few words)
- Repetitive—repeating phrases over
- Inappropriate speech—speech which makes little sense
- Echolalia—repeating the vocalizations of another
- Scripting—repeating lines from a movie or TV show over and over

Social Problems:
- Does not understand typical social boundaries or behavior in social situations

- Decreased imaginary and pretend play
- Extremely hyperactive or underactive
- Extreme tantrums—uncontrollable
- Tunes others out, plays by self
- Frequently does not notice someone entering the room
- Inappropriate playing with toys or prefers objects that are not toys
- Poor eye contact
- Lack of fear in dangerous situations (climbing on shelves)
- Often does not return a happy smile from parents
- Difficulty with transitions (could be location or activity transitions)

Sensory Problems:
- Unusual pain tolerance
- Avoids close contact or makes unusually close contact (looks into face)
- Frequently annoyed by certain sensations such as clothing tags, wearing shoes, and/or avoids or seeks out certain textures (sand, carpeting, grass)
- Bothered by large noisy, crowds
- Sensory seeking—requires deep pressure squeezing, hugging, and/or massage

Movement Problems:
- Self-stimulating behaviors (known as "stimming"; i.e. hand flapping, repetitive movements, lining up objects)
- Self-restricted diet (eats only chicken nuggets)
- Unusually aggressive or self-injurious behaviors (head banging, bites self)
- Obsessed with routines (avoids change)
- Obsession with spinning objects

3. And from the National Autism Association—warning signs your child may have autism:

- Little or no eye contact
- Does not respond to name by 12 months
- Does not babble or coo by 12 months
- Does not gesture or point by 12 months
- Does not say single words by 16 months
- Has ANY loss of ANY language or social skills at ANY age

4. Children who are at risk (particularly those whose parents have auto-immune conditions or siblings on the spectrum) should be watched very closely for any of the symptoms listed above.

5. A child with autism will often experience sensory overload; they will cover their ears to sounds which overwhelm them, cover their eyes or look away from painful visual impressions, and may self-limit their diet or attempt to taste non-food items to avoid or satiate acute tastes.

6. Many kids who are eventually diagnosed with autism had at the beginning some evidence of hypersensitivities, focused around auditory, tactile, and vestibular (body position and movement) inputs. Others may show no reaction to auditory, tactile, and vestibular inputs due to hypotonia (low muscle tone and the inability to respond with movement).

7. For an autistic child already in the first sensory motor phase, the individual relationship with a key person, usually the mother, fails to appear, and the child's attention is directed mainly towards the spatial world.

—Bob Woodward and Dr. Marga Hogenboom,
Autism: A Holistic Approach

8. Children with Asperger's syndrome may not display any real challenges until third or fourth grade, when organizing school assignments becomes more complicated, and the children start changing classrooms. Your son may be frustrated with school, or fall behind because of his lack of organizational skills, and you may find yourself irritated with what looks like a lack of effort. A teacher may also notice that something is amiss. You may be noticing problems in the social skills area, or hear from the school about problems during recess or during PE, where athletic and social skills are required. If you suspect that your child has Asperger's syndrome, and you've ruled out distractions like bad chemistry with the teacher or a social issue, your best recourse is to have the child tested for an Autism Spectrum Disorder (ASD).

9. If your pediatrician isn't seeing what you see, don't wait for him/her to come around. If your child is under the age of three, contact your state's early childhood intervention program and ask for an evaluation. You can also visit a developmental pediatrician or a clinical psychologist trained in diagnosing ASD.

—Anissa Ryland, Director, Thoughtful House Center for Children

10. Even if your family pediatrician suspects an ASD, it's a good idea to bring your child to a professional who specializes in diagnosing ASDs. Your pediatrician can recommend a specialist, or you can find one through your local hospital, school district, university, or state agency that specializes in ASDs.

—Karen Siff Exkorn, *The Autism Sourcebook*

CHAPTER 2

Welcome to the Club Nobody Wants to Join

11. There are certain historical events that greatly impact the world, and all people grieve and acknowledge together the feelings they share. Events such as the terrorist attacks on 9/11, or the day that President John F. Kennedy was assassinated, or the day that Princess Diana was killed in a car accident in Paris; you never forget where you were when you found out about these events. The day you receive the news of your child's diagnosis is just as traumatic; the only difference is, no one else is sharing your pain. The people you pass on the street have the same life they had an hour ago, but yours has changed forever.

—Chantal Sicile-Kira, www.chantalsicile-kira.com

12. As a parent, you did not choose to have a boy with autism. However, you *can* choose how you are going to react and what you are going to do about it. The first step is to acknowledge the emotions you are feeling. Realize that all parents go through these emotions—they are real and unavoidable. These emotions have been likened to the five stages of grief that a person goes through when faced with the death of a loved one. In this case, your son is still here, but what you are mourning is the loss of your expectations, of everything you had hoped and dreamed for with the birth of your son. The second step is learning all you can to help your child recover or reach his full potential.

—Chantal Sicile-Kira, www.chantalsicile-kira.com

13. Once you have determined that your child's development and be-havior profile contains autistic manifestations and features, you will be guided (by a variety of well-intentioned and well-meaning pro-fessionals or parents) onto the "Autism Superhighway." Do not al-low yourself to journey down the road marked CURE. Instead, travel down the road toward RECOVERY. The journey to recovery will not be a sprint but a marathon. There will be times when the road is smooth and straight and times when there will be curves, dead ends, and detours. Find yourself a developmental pediatrician or another professional who is willing to be your guide and GPS system. Avoid cookie-cutter approaches, interventions, and action plans. Instead, let your child's unique and individual profile guide you on this journey.

—Dr. Mark Freilich, Total Kids Developmental

Pediatric Resources, New York City

14. Early intervention is the best intervention, so speed is of the essence. Contact the nearest good early-intervention program, which will no doubt have a waiting list. Get on it no matter how long it is; the waits are frequently shorter than predicted. Stress that your child is under the age of three, as younger children are given priority.

15. Solicit help from friends and family; a strong support system can be of enormous help.

16. Contact the local chapters of the Autism Society of America (ASA), the National Autism Association (NAA), and Talk About Curing Autism (TACA), and find parents to connect with and learn from. They can share information about professionals and schools in the area. Professionals are often restricted when it comes to the information they can share.

17. Start a crash course of self-education—you need to become an autism expert now. Check your resources: be careful where you get your information, as anybody can put up a website or self-publish a book. There is a great deal of information, but start by subscribing to *The Advocate, Spectrum Magazine, The Autism File,* and the *ARRI Quarterly.*

18. As you move forward in your treatments, school selection, and other endeavors, do not become wedded to any one institution or individual. Things will change with your child over time and you will need to monitor and adjust programs and individuals accordingly. Be flexible and constantly seek improvements.

19. Accept and love your child for who he is. Rather than focusing on how your autistic child is different from other children and what he or she is "missing," focus on what makes your child happy. Enjoy your kid's special quirks, celebrate small successes, and stop comparing your child to others—developmentally challenged or not.

—Reprinted with permission from Helpguide.org. See www.helpguide.org/mental/autism_help.htm for additional resources and support.

20. Be patient and optimistic. It's impossible to predict the course of an autism spectrum disorder. Don't jump to conclusions about what life is going to be like for your child. Like everyone else, people with autism have an entire lifetime to grow and develop their abilities.

—Reprinted with permission from Helpguide.org. See www.helpguide.org/mental/autism_help.htm for additional resources and support.

21. Don't believe everything you read on the Internet, especially the stuff that blames you as a parent for your child's condition. It's not your fault; it never was, and it never will be.

—Donna Satterlee Ross and Kelly Ann Jolly, *That's Life with Autism*

22. Likewise, stay away from anyone offering a "cure," or anyone who professes that his or her method will work for everyone with an ASD.

23. Just because one professional doesn't have an answer doesn't mean the next won't. Talk to as many people as possible. Educate yourself. Keep asking questions. The answer may be out there, and it's up to you to find it.

—Judith Chinitz, MS, MS, CNC, author of *We Band of Mothers*

24. Don't ignore your inner parent voice. If you think a professional is off-base, don't dismiss your instinct because you're "just" a parent, and he or she is a highly esteemed professional. Get another opinion.

—Jane Johnson, Managing Director, Autism Research Institute

25. If you keep trying you may have only a .001 percent chance of helping your child—but that's still more than the 0 percent chance they'll have if you give up.

Judith Chinitz, MS, MS, CNC, author of *We Band of Mothers*

26. Please don't make the mistake of getting so caught up with what caused your child's ASD that you miss out on getting immediate treatment for your child. As much as you may want to find the reason why your child has an ASD, it's important that you attend to what's really important right now.

—Karen Siff Exkorn, *The Autism Sourcebook*

27. The earlier a child begins treatment, preferably as soon as the first sign of autism is noticed, the easier treatment can be, and the more rapid the recovery or improvement.

—Julie A. Buckley, MD, *Healing our Autistic Children*

28. Parents need to know at the outset that the complexity of ASD means that diagnostics and treatment are neither easy nor quick. A great deal of devotion, time, patience, and hard work is required; the strains upon economic and emotional resources may be great.

—Jaquelyn McCandless, *Children with Starving Brains*

29. One must modify one's expectations. Expecting too much at one go is not advisable. Set small goals for the autistic child, which he or she is able to achieve.

> —Instah.com, "The 10 Ways of Dealing with Autistic Children";
> www.instah.com/children-health/top-10-ways-of-
> dealing-with-autistic-children/

30. As soon as you can cope, start advocating in the community. Real change only comes about when people make it happen.

> —Casey van der Grient; www.autism-resources.com
> /advice-to-parents.html

....

Diagnosis and Evaluation—Formation

Well, your son has been diagnosed with autism. He is now a child with autism, not autistic. Remember that distinction, because if you have autism, you can improve. If you are autistic, that is who you are. Now pick yourself up; there is much to be done. And remember—you are now in a club with others. None of us wanted to be here, but here we are, together. You are not alone. Read on.

Chapter 3

About the Diagnosis

31. There are some medical problems that can be mistaken for autism, and diagnosing and treating these early is a good idea. The usual suspects include seizure disorders, including Rett and Landau-Kleffner, mitochondrial disorders, and stroke in utero, among others.

—Tara Marshall

32. The first step toward obtaining assistance for your son is getting a diagnosis of autism. Many parents have a hard time with this, since a child doesn't always display the behaviors they are concerned about during a doctor's appointment. Recording your son's behavior and showing it to the doctor can be extremely helpful.

33. A diagnosis of Pervasive Development Disorder–Not Otherwise Specified (PDD-NOS) in a young child (toddler) is likely to change over time. Frequently it leads to a full autism diagnosis, particularly without early intervention. This being the case, proceed as if you have received an autism diagnosis.

34. Specialists sometimes choose PDD-NOS instead of an autism diagnosis because they think the "a-word" frightens parents. Don't be afraid of the label, because it will help you get the services you need.

35. Individuals with Asperger's syndrome (AS) may escape into their imaginations, in some cases creating an entire imaginary world that is more hospitable than the one in which they find themselves. In such cases, the children simply appear creative or imaginative, and few suspect AS.

> —Jennifer Copley, "Girls with Asperger's Syndrome: Gender Differences in Behavior and Social Interaction," April 4, 2008, www.suite101.com/content/girls-with-aspergers-syndrome-a49866#ixzz0y1Wlj7CG

36. Diagnoses you may receive:

- Autism spectrum disorder.
- Asperger's syndrome—Social skills are the issue.
- Childhood disintegrative disorder—Learning skills totally disintegrate, including toileting; includes low IQ and mental retardation.
- Rett syndrome—More common in girls, 1 in every 10,000 to 15,000. Includes autism symptoms along with motor coordination problems; onset at 6 to 18 months.
- Pervasive developmental disorder–not otherwise specified (PDD-NOS)—Child does not meet sufficient criteria for diagnosis of autism or Asperger's. Frequently children are initially diagnosed with PDD-NOS and then move to autism.

CHAPTER 4

Which Evaluations to Get, and How to Get Them

37. For early intervention services, if a child is under the age of three, call your local early intervention agency. Check your state's Developmental Disability Agency for more information at www.ddrcco.com/states.htm.

38. For special education services, if a child is three or older, contact the local school district.

39. Before services can be provided, it might be necessary to complete further assessments and evaluations. These might include:
- An unstructured diagnostic play session
- A developmental evaluation
- A speech-language assessment
- A parent interview
- An evaluation of current behavior
- An evaluation of adaptive or real-life skills
- A psychological evaluation
- A psychosocial evaluation
- Autism Diagnostic Observation Scale (ADOS)
- Autism Diagnostic Review/Autism Rating Scale (ADI-R)
- Childhood Autism Rating Scale (CARS)
- Speech
- Occupational

40. Remember: You have the right to request private evaluations each year if your son is not making progress.

41. Be sure that evaluators fully assess your perspective and your experiences of your child. The best results and recommendations from evaluations are based on well-validated and/or standardized assessment tools, a complete psychosocial history, parent report, and clinical observations of the child's interactions with peers, family members, and the evaluator.

—Lauren Tobing-Puente, PhD, Licensed Psychologist,
www.drtobingpuente.com

42. Before patients and physicians can agree on the best treatment decisions, a good diagnosis is critical. Many treatment options are available, and I have found that most of these children need many kinds of therapy, some applied simultaneously and some sequentially, to optimize the outcome.

—Jaquelyn McCandless, *Children with Starving Brains*

43. Once your son turns three, any therapies implemented by the state may be assumed by the public school system.

44. To garner the highest amount of services for your child, do not shy away from an autism diagnosis/label. If your son is on the border of autism and "high-functioning," go for the full autism diagnosis— you will receive more hours of therapy, and the diagnosis can always be adjusted later with improvement. Additionally, if your son is on the autism/mental retardation (MR) border, work to get the autism label—again, the level and amount of therapy is superior, given perceived better outcomes for autism over MR.

SECTION 3

....

Education—Planning a Siege

Your son's diagnosis is complete. You have marshaled your forces and organized yourself. Now heed the words of Sun Tzu:

> Plan for what is difficult while it is easy; do what is great while it is small. The most difficult things in the world must be done while they are still easy; the greatest things in the world must be done while they are still small. For this reason sages never do what is great, and this is why they can achieve greatness.

CHAPTER 5

IDEA: Your Child's Rights on the Battleground

45. Under the Individuals with Disabilities Education Act (IDEA), services such as speech therapy, occupational therapy, vision therapy, and behavioral therapy can be provided to the child by the school district, on the condition that it has been decided that it needs to be a part of the student's individualized program at an Individual Education Program (IEP) team meeting, and written into the IEP. Parents need to inform themselves about the school district they are in, the quality of the services, their rights, and which professional in the area is the best to provide assessments of your child.

—Chantal Sicile-Kira, www.chantalsicile-kira.com

46. IDEA was passed in 1990 and is designed to provide kids with learning disabilities an *appropriate* education in the least restrictive environment possible. Parents are to be partners in choosing the best education fit. To do this, parents need to become familiar with the law so they know their rights and what services are available for their children.

47. Parent rights under IDEA include the right to ask for an evaluation of your child at any time and the right to be part of the team deciding what special education services and therapies will be provided to your child.

48. IDEA provides for your child to have an Individualized Education Plan (IEP) designed for his specific needs; for example, how much occupational, physical, and speech therapy will be provided.

49. The specific services to be provided are decided at the annual IEP meeting, which includes yourself, your son's teachers, various school representatives, and a parent representative. You can bring your own specialists and support folks to help you in any way (moral support, reminders, etc.).

50. It's best to consult with a specialized education attorney before attending the meeting.

51. Bring a copy of the law with you to review prior to sitting down at the meeting. It's also important to bring along any other helpful documentation. Many times, they (the state team) will incorporate what you give them.

52. Should your son not progress, you have the right to question the plan and request an IEP meeting at any time to reassess the services and service levels (number of sessions) provided.

53. If there is a conflict with the educators, you have the right to have your son reevaluated. In this case, you may want to seek out a private evaluation, which can cost from a few hundred to a few thousand dollars. If you have a Medicaid waiver, you may be able to get a free outside evaluation (or at least a discounted one). Depending on where you live, it could take a while to get an appointment, so call as early as possible.

54. Should you not come to an agreement with your son's school system, you do have the right to a due process hearing where an administrative officer or judge rules. Should it come to this, you will require the services of a lawyer. Again, it's best to have an attorney (specializing in education law) in advance of this eventuality, if at all possible.

55. The U.S. Department of Education has information about federal laws and state laws. Every state has a Protection and Advocacy office which can provide you with free information in regard to your child's rights under special education. Most offices provide these laws and your rights in simple language for the layperson, in English as well as in different languages.

56. What's the big IDEA? It's important to know that IDEA is in effect for your child until he graduates from high school, or at least until he reaches the age of twenty-one; after this point, services are provided on a state-by-state basis. Under IDEA, every child is entitled to a Free and Appropriate Public Education (FAPE), regardless of disability. In this context, the U.S. Supreme Court has taken *appropriate* to mean that the program "must be reasonably calculated to provide educational benefit to the individual child." In addition, under IDEA, all children are to be placed in the *least* restrictive environment possible. Remember: Special education is a service, and *not* a place.

57. Here are the key parental rights under IDEA to remember:

- Parents have the right to be informed and knowledgeable about all actions taken on behalf of their child.
- Parents have the right to participate in all meetings regarding evaluation and placement.
- Parental consent is required for evaluation and placement.
- Parents have the right to challenge educational decisions through due process procedures.

58. The related services your son may be entitled to include:

- Speech therapy
- Occupational therapy
- Counseling
- Nursing services—medication administration
- Transportation
- Paraprofessional—health and/or transportation para

59. Tips for Achieving the Least Restrictive Environment for Your Child

by Timothy A. Adams, Esq. and Lynne Arnold, MA

- Don't allow your child to lose out on the benefits of being educated alongside typically developing peers. The least restrictive environment (LRE) is a fundamental requirement of IDEA (Individuals with Disabilities Education Act): *To the maximum extent appropriate, children with disabilities, including children in public or private institutions or other care facilities, are educated with children who are not disabled, and special classes, separate schooling, or other removal of children with disabilities from the regular educational environment occurs only when the nature or severity of the disability of a child is such that education in regular classes with the use of supplementary aids and services cannot be achieved satisfactorily.* 20 USC § 1412(a)(5)

- Get an independent educational evaluation (IEE) of your child's needs. This can be done by a behaviorist or psychologist with educational experience who observes your child at school and/or at any placement proposed by your school district. This professional can provide a third-party, objective recommendation on the appropriate placement as well as the accommodations and modifications that are necessary for your child to succeed.

- Remember that general education is the default placement. Before offering a more restrictive environment, the school district must consider what supplementary supports and services, accommodations or modifications would allow the child to be successful in a general education setting.

- Don't be afraid to ask "why?" It's the school district's job to explain to you why its placement offer is the LRE for your child. The IEP team must review the continuum of placement options before determining which one is the LRE for your child. As the parent, you're the most important member of that team. Be sure to personally observe any proposed placement and consider bringing an independent evaluator with you.

- Ask the IEP team to explain each time segment of your child's school day that has been designated as "inclusion" or "mainstreaming." Make sure that any time your child's IEP says he will spend among typical peers is meaningful. Otherwise for example, your child's inclusion time during lunch may only mean that your child is in the cafeteria at the same time as the regular education children. Your child may be restricted to a special table and/or there is no attempt to facilitate his interaction with general education students.

- Consider the benefits of your child's exposure to same-aged peers who are modeling age-appropriate language, skills, and abilities. Children learn from each other and imitate each other. Inclusion can make a big difference for a child both academically and socially, and eventually determine if the child will be on track for a certificate or diploma upon high school graduation.

- Deconstruct your child's challenges in a goal-oriented framework. What are the specific barriers to your child being successful in a regular education placement? Break down each challenge into goals—then brainstorm on what accommodations, modifications and behavioral supports are necessary for your child to achieve greater independence in the classroom.

- Don't accept excuses that general education with an aide is more restrictive than a special education classroom. By definition, LRE is determined by the child's exposure to his typically developing peers. If an aide is keeping a child from his peers, that's a training and supervision issue, not an appropriate rationale to keep a child segregated in a special education classroom.

- Ask the IEP team about the implications of various placements. If the district says your child's needs will be best met in a special education classroom, make sure you understand the specifics of those supposed advantages. For example, although a special day class will typically have a higher ratio of teachers/aides to children, it's not a matter of simple math. Some aides may already be assigned to provide 1:1 help to specific children and overall, the class may include children whose exceptional needs would skew the actual ratio throughout the school day. Also, the number of the children in the classroom can widely fluctuate throughout the school year.

- Don't let unaddressed problems become an excuse for removing your child from a general education classroom. For example, if a child is disruptive, determine a plan for reducing and eliminating the problem behaviors, which often includes developing a behavior plan. It's an absolute inequity for an IEP team to simply move a disruption into a special education classroom. If your child's behavior is disruptive, why is it unacceptable for the general education classmates, but reasonable for the special education classmates to experience?

- Don't allow your child's right to an *individualized* education program to be solely determined by the district's existing structure for special education placement. For example, districts often tell parents that a particular classroom or program requires a certain testing score or other subjective criteria. Just because your child doesn't fit neatly into their existing programs doesn't lessen their obligation under state and federal laws to meet his educational needs.

- If not now, when? Now is the best time to determine how a child can gain educational benefit from inclusion. If the IEP team is not offering inclusion, what are their reasons? If the district is refusing to provide the least restrictive environment, they must provide Prior Written Notice [34 CFR §300.503(a)] which includes a description of their refusal, the reasons for that refusal, description of factors considered in their refusal, explanation of alternative choices, any other reasons for their refusal, resources for the parent to understand Part B of the IDEA and a copy of the parents' procedural rights.

CHAPTER 6

Individualized Education Program (IEP): Your Child's Weapons

60. When speaking to your son's Board of Education (BOE), remember the phrase, "appropriate education." Your son is entitled by the Individuals with Disabilities Education Act (IDEA) to a free appropriate public education. If your BOE cannot provide one, they must cover the cost of an APPROPRIATE private school. Appropriate does not mean best! Keep this in mind. *The Supreme Court interprets an appropriate education plan as one that "must be reasonably calculated to provide educational benefit to the individual child."*

61. Remember, services are expensive, and, because of financial pressures, your state would prefer to offer as little as possible—so be prepared to fight.

62. Should you believe a private school is the best option, and you'll miss the $60,000 to $100,000 they cost, you will need an education lawyer. EDUCATION LAWYER. Not Uncle Steve or your next-door neighbor who happens to be an attorney. For this you need a specialist. Ask your target school, as they likely have a list of lawyers other parents use. Interview a few and choose the one you like, and ask for parent references!

63. Be aware that parents have a lot of power. Don't wait for two months to check in for results. If something is not resolved quickly, work on it. Teachers don't always have as much leverage as you think. You may be able to help your child's teacher resolve something much faster. Work as a team.

—Autism and PDD Support Network; www.autism-pdd.net/autism-tips.html

64. You and the district will have to come up with an Individual Education Plan (IEP). To prepare, read *The Complete IEP Guide: How to Advocate for Your Special Ed Child* by attorney Lawrence Siegel, and talk to parents already in the school system you are targeting to learn about what they have experienced.

65. Take the first step. Call the school district to find out the process for requesting an evaluation and an individualized education plan (IEP). The IEP, which is required by federal law, is the document that will guide teachers as they work with your child. All school districts operate differently when it comes to the IEP process.

—Patti Ghezzi, SchoolFamily.com,
www.schoolfamily.com/school-family-articles/
article/10685-help-your-autistic-child-succeed-in-school

66. Focus on what you're legally entitled to. By studying local, state, and federal laws, you will know going in what your district can do to help your child. Don't waste time arguing for services that are not indicated by the IEP.

—Patti Ghezzi, SchoolFamily.com,
www.schoolfamily.com/school-family-articles/
article/10685-help-your-autistic-child-succeed-in-school

67. Don't make assumptions. Small schools can offer excellent services, and large schools can offer poor services. Schools in rural areas can be enlightened. Schools in suburban districts can be stuck in outdated methods. Get to know your child's IEP team members, and keep an open mind. Sometimes teachers need to be educated about autism and are open to learning more if it means helping your child.

—Patti Ghezzi, SchoolFamily.com,
www.schoolfamily.com/school-family-articles
/article/10685-help-your-autistic-child-succeed-in-school

68. Bring up your child's sensory needs. "Address sensory issues promptly," Ellen Notbohm says. "If he can't tolerate being in his own skin, how is he going to learn?" Notbohm likens the experience an autistic child has in a classroom to being on a roller coaster; it's an intense assault on the senses. "In the middle of all that, a child is asked to focus on schoolwork," she says.

—Patti Ghezzi, SchoolFamily.com,
www.schoolfamily.com/school-family-articles
/article/10685-help-your-autistic-child-succeed-in-school

69. Teachers who work with autistic children need to understand associative thought patterns. An autistic child will often use a word in an inappropriate manner. Sometimes these uses have a logical associative meaning and other times they don't.

—Temple Grandin, PhD, *Thinking in Pictures*

70. Be optimistic. Stories of battles between parents and teachers over education for a special needs child are common, but there are many success stories.

—Patti Ghezzi, SchoolFamily.com,
www.schoolfamily.com/school-family-articles
/article/10685-help-your-autistic-child-succeed-in-school

71. If you feel that decisions are being made without you, call and ask to be included in discussions. You can suggest a "pre-IEP" meeting to talk about some of your ideas and what your goals and the goals of your child are. This is especially helpful for meetings that involve therapists and/or both special and general education staff. By talking before the meeting with the specific people who are responsible for your areas of concern, you can structure the formal meeting so it goes smoothly and so the entire group can sign off with only one meeting.

—Autism and PDD Support Network;
www.autism-pdd.net/autism-tips.html

72. Encourage a work ethic at home. Put value on those traits that promote success in school: responsibility, consequences for behavior, organization, and punctuality. Jobs at home translate into expectations. A sense of cooperation and self-worth follow.

—Autism and PDD Support Network;
www.autism-pdd.net/autism-tips.html

CHAPTER 7

Finding the Right School

73. When looking at schools, focus on the right educational *and* therapeutic environment for your son. The right educational program in an overcrowded, busy school will not help your son in the long run if he has significant sensory issues. A smaller, soothing class might accomplish more than the educational program itself. Overall, choose the environment that will allow your son to function at his best.

74. Consider moving to another state. Some states spend a greater percentage of their budgets on social services and thus have more services available. These states tend to have a higher percentage of children with autism as well, so there are more parents to network with and likely more specialized schools. Put politics aside, because you need all the help you can get; seek out those states friendliest to the "autism family." Easter Seals has compiled a list titled State Autism Profiles: www.easterseals.com/site/_autism_state_profiles. Check it out and see where your state ranks.

75. In school, your son's class should have almost as many teachers and assistants as kids. If he is high-functioning end of the spectrum, focus on mainstreaming and having typical peer interactions. If on the severe end of the spectrum, focus on a high teacher-student ratio and large amounts of therapy time.

76. View the lists of special needs that a school can meet with a certain amount of skepticism: Make sure the school addresses the difficulties of the conditions, and doesn't just contain them, or think they can cope because they "had a student with this diagnosis a year or so back." Ensure that the staff receives training in their students' particular difficulties. Go for a school or classroom placement which offers the right experience.

—Oaasis Information Sheet: Finding a Special Needs School/Home Learning, www.oaasis.co.uk/documents/Info_Sheets /Finding_A_Special_Needs_School

77. Nothing is as important as making a personal visit on a normal working day to a short-list of several schools. Do not take your child with you on these preliminary informal trips; he may become excited, confused, or agitated, especially if he visits several in a short span of time.

—Oaasis Information Sheet: Finding a Special Needs School/Home Learning, www.oaasis.co.uk/documents/Info_Sheets /Finding_A_Special_Needs_School

78. Don't ignore intuitive thoughts. If everything looks wonderful but you just don't feel that a school is right for your child, then listen to yourself. Remember: People can thrive in the most outlandish of places and unkempt of homes; genuine affection, enthusiasm, patience, concern, and knowledgeable understanding from staff rate far higher than fresh coats of paint and new curtains.

—Oaasis Information Sheet: Independent Special Schools— What to Look For, www.oaasis.co.uk/documents/Info_Sheets /Independent_Special_Schools_What_To_Look_For

79. It is often an educational goal for parents and professionals for a child to be mainstreamed. While an important goal, it is more important to consider your child's feelings of competence in these settings. Typical role models can be good, but the reality is that children's interactions are full of innuendo. Academically, your child may be able to keep up with a mainstream class, but socially, he or she is likely lagging behind. Ask yourself: Are these role models providing positive experiences for my child, or is my child feeling bullied, isolated, or incompetent in that environment?

—Laura Hynes, LMSW, RDI® Program Certified Consultant,
www.extraordinaryminds.org

80. Consider choosing a school in which your child will not be noticeably more "peculiar" than everyone else; children are harsh critics. Children on the spectrum will not pick up typical behavior by observation; it will need to be formally taught to them.

81. Children who attend learning-disabled schools are often more accepting of differences in others; even if they are simply dyslexic, they often place less value on conformity.

82. Some questions to ask when you visit a recommended program:

- What is the educational philosophy of the program (ABA, DIR, TEAACH)?
- What is the class size and ratio to teachers/teaching assistants?
- How long has the school been using the current program (ABA, DIR, etc.)?
- How do the nonverbal kids communicate?
- What kind of success has the program had (i.e., kids moving to less-restrictive classes)?
- What programs are offered to parents?
- How long has the teacher taught at this school?
- What is their experience with kids with autism?
- How are related services provided?
- What services are currently being provided to students in the class?
- Does the school have a consultant or supervisor certified in the particular philosophy?
- Does the consultant/supervisor conduct ongoing training for school staff?
- What is the age makeup of the class? (There can only be a three-year age span in each class.)
- Where do the special education kids have lunch and recreation?
- Are there inclusion opportunities?
- How does the staff handle behavioral issues and/or self-injurious behaviors?
- What types of reinforcers are used at the school?
- Is medical staff available at the school?

Don't forget to observe a class and take copious notes!

83. It is illegal for a school to tell parents that their child cannot come back to school unless on medication!

84. Parents will need a doctor note indicating what services are needed for their child, along with an indication of the diagnosis.

School Design and Environments
Tips by Cathy Purple Cherry, AIA, LEED AP

- Consideration should be given to the placement of windows within each classroom. If windows are held higher such that when students are sitting down and learning they cannot see individuals and movement outside, this will help reduce distraction while still allowing for natural light. Also, the amount of glass within the entry door to each classroom should be minimized, again to reduce the opportunity to see movement outside of the learning environment.
- The heating and cooling system should be designed so that the temperature in each classroom can be controlled separately. This will allow the teacher to create the most comfortable environment for his or her students.
- Appropriate lighting should be selected to eliminate glare and flickering movement.
- Each classroom should be ideally sound-isolated from the adjacent spaces. This helps reduce or eliminate noise transfer.

- Generally, all schools should be durable due to the number of students that use these buildings. The durability of selected materials is also a consideration for the life cycle of the school. Within the spectrum, explosive issues, such as intermittent explosive disorder or bipolar, can also co-habitat with ASD. Further, when the autistic child experiences puberty, their physical strength can be used in ways not expected even by them. The need, therefore, exists to use durable materials in these school settings.

- At times, students with ASD also require time-out rooms to allow the child or teen to regain self-control during periods of outburst. These time-out rooms must be durable and ideally sound-isolated. Most important, these spaces should be separated from the public areas of the school so as to provide the isolated child with greater dignity. The sense of shame or guilt that the secluded student feels when friends walk by can be huge. In addition, the distractions that occur to the others in the adjacent social hub or corridor are great. The solution to this is to locate the room for privacy. This further removes the audience from the individual that at times can be stimulating, and removes the disruption from others in adjacent spaces.

- On the other hand, when hard and smooth materials are used for durability, frequently acoustics can become an issue. It is so important to manage the acoustics of the learning environments for children with ASD, as loud noises can be both distracting as well as disturbing. Sensory bombardment and inappropriate noises can trigger inappropriate actions. General sound levels as well as white noise can further cause learning problems for individuals with auditory issues. White noise from mechanical and electrical systems can also interfere with a child's ability to properly process sound. Architectural applications that can assist in managing some levels of sound include installation of sound-absorption materials as wall or ceiling panels, installing carpet in selected areas, placing rubber balls on the bottom of furniture legs, hanging baffles and banners within the classroom, utilizing fabrics on furniture, and installing airflow silencers.

- Children with ASD can also respond differently than typically developing peers to colors and patterns. Those with visual sensitivities must be considered when selecting finish applications in the school environment. Colors, patterns, and contrast can create problems with sustained attention. At times, minimizing the offending stimuli can help improve the individual's ability to perform in other areas.

- Playground areas can provide ASD students the opportunity to explore social contact as well as places to be left alone. Security is important to assist in defining boundaries and providing safe playground environments. Playground areas can be designed to stimulate and provide physical opportunities for ASD children with gross motor skill challenges; wider openings between play structures can allow for easy access and support personal space needs; equipment can be designed to be sensory-rich; hard-scaped areas should be covered with rubberized materials for safety; ramps can connect to structures and climbing equipment can be made lower to permit the physically-challenged opportunities to participate in play activity; outdoor activities such as landscaping and digging can provide physical challenges and assist in developing vocational skills for high school students; landscaped paths can help define edges; brightly colored equipment can provide sensory stimulation; and secluded areas can provide safe distances from people whose voices and activities could overstimulate.

- Further, ASD students often have difficulty with a clear understanding of the personal space requirements between themselves and other individuals. This misunderstanding of the necessary personal space needed between two individuals can lead to intense conflict. As children, we learned how to interact with others, to take turns, and to understand the distance we should stand away from people depending upon our familiarity with them. We also learned what to do or how to react when others entered our personal space. Autistic children are not aware of this social dance. They can frequently come too close to other individuals, causing an invasion of privacy and true discomfort. This direct contact can lead to a basic feeling of disrespect or, in the extreme, an explosive event.

- Finally, the most exciting change to the classroom environments for ASD children is the development of innovative technology and multimedia. These creative tools have rapidly accelerated the learning and communication abilities of children with autism. By implementing interactive technology, school programs can successfully support collaboration, communication and engaged learning.

CHAPTER 8

Communicating with the School

85. Communication: The most important thing to do is to establish open communication. Try to be nonthreatening. You can make friends and get what you need.

—Autism and PDD Support Network;
www.autism-pdd.net/autism-tips.html

86. But if making friends doesn't work, prepare to fight!

87. Look at yourself closely to identify habits or attitudes that interfere with effective communication or your being taken seriously.

—Autism and PDD Support Network;
www.autism-pdd.net/autism-tips.html

88. Be sure to communicate any concerns or ideas right away, over the phone or with a note, while the discussion can be relatively casual. By communicating early, you can avoid becoming angry and frustrated; by intervening early, you can avoid a situation growing into a bigger problem or crisis.

—Autism and PDD Support Network;
www.autism-pdd.net/autism-tips.html

89. Consider your options. When you're having a contentious experience with your child's teacher, or when you think your child needs more than the school will be able to provide, look into private therapy, which might be covered by insurance. If you aren't able to access services your child is entitled to, consider hiring an advocate or special education attorney to help you work with the school. Be the squeaky wheel that gets the grease.

—Patti Ghezzi, SchoolFamily.com,
www.schoolfamily.com/school-family-articles
/article/10685-help-your-autistic-child-succeed-in-school

90. Whether a child with autism is in elementary, middle, or high school, the first step to fostering support begins with parents meeting with teachers and school leaders. Every public school is legally required to offer all students special services, and therefore, the earlier parents can meet with the school, the more tailored the program can be made for your autistic child.

—Grace Chen, "5 Tips for Helping Your Autistic Child Excel in Public Schools," www.publicschoolreview.com/articles/88

91. As autism rates are soaring across the country, many schools are creating programs, classes, and resources specifically for students with autism. If the school does not offer these resources, ask leaders if any nearby cooperating county/district schools provide autism-specific support.

> —Grace Chen, "5 Tips for Helping Your Autistic Child Excel in Public Schools," www.publicschoolreview.com/articles/88

92. When meeting with the teachers and staff, find out how much experience the teachers have with autistic students. This is an opportunity for parents to seek out answers to all relevant questions that will impact their child's upcoming academic year. Additionally, parents have a moral obligation to inform the teachers of any behavioral concerns or issues relating to their child.

> —Grace Chen, "5 Tips for Helping Your Autistic Child Excel in Public Schools," www.publicschoolreview.com/articles/88

93. As autistic children struggle with learning appropriate social behaviors, many exhibit occasional outbursts, physical tendencies/quirks, inappropriate speech/comments, and so forth. If this is part of a child's behavioral pattern, then the parent must honestly and truthfully disclose this information. The more informed the teachers are, the better they can prepare for the child.

> —Grace Chen, "5 Tips for Helping Your Autistic Child Excel in Public Schools," www.publicschoolreview.com/articles/88

94. When meeting with teachers, parents should set up a clear and agreeable communication pattern. As students with autism often exhibit unexpected behavior, outbursts, or other tendencies, parents and teachers must be able to quickly contact one another in the case of an urgent need or emergency.

> —Grace Chen, "5 Tips for Helping Your Autistic Child Excel in Public Schools," www.publicschoolreview.com/articles/88

95. Considering that many autistic students struggle with organizational skills, teachers and parents can set up a communication plan so that parents are informed of all assignments and upcoming assessments. A positive pattern of communication might include asking the teacher to e-mail the parent each day with a quick summary of homework and upcoming quizzes or tests. Or, on the other hand, if the child needs less support, then an alternative plan could involve the parent calling or e-mailing the teacher when a concern arises. By informing the teacher(s) of a child's needs and abilities, the parent can help boost the ease of their child's education and development by creating a regular routine of dialogue with their child's teacher(s).

—Grace Chen, "5 Tips for Helping Your Autistic Child Excel in Public Schools," www.publicschoolreview.com/articles/88

96. In addition to establishing and maintaining a routine and plan for communicating with a child's teacher, parents must also reinforce routines at home. As autistic children and adults often struggle with issues of high anxiety and worry, parents can help assuage feelings of angst by adhering to a daily program and regimen.

—Grace Chen, "5 Tips for Helping Your Autistic Child Excel in Public Schools," www.publicschoolreview.com/articles/88

97. Although more schools are providing teachers with training for special-needs and autistic children, not all teachers are fully informed on the needs and demands of this spectrum. Despite this, parents need to have a respectful and trusting relationship with their child's teacher. If a teacher observes some form of behavior or expresses a concern, parents need to remind themselves not to take this feedback personally. Concerns from teachers that involve moving a child to a lower or higher class, or providing a child with appropriate discipline, should be discussed openly with a parent.

—Grace Chen, "5 Tips for Helping Your Autistic Child Excel in Public Schools," www.publicschoolreview.com/articles/88

98. While parents need to respect a teacher's expertise and feedback, moms and dads should also keep in mind that they have the right to ask questions and request administrator intervention if they are concerned about their child's teacher. If, for any reason, parents feel uncomfortable with a teacher's actions, responses, or communication with their autistic child, they can begin by first speaking respectfully with the teacher. If this is not an effective conversation, then parents always reserve the right to advocate for their child by speaking with another school leader. Ultimately, parents want to strive to maintain a positive, honest, and cooperative relationship with school leaders and staff.

—Grace Chen, "5 Tips for Helping Your Autistic Child Excel in Public Schools," www.publicschoolreview.com/articles/88

99. Write letters or make calls to say thank-you when things are going well. It's always a good idea to let educators know about successes, especially those that occur outside of school. For really successful occurrences, send a copy of your letter to the principal or supervisor, so he or she will also know what a great job your child's teacher is doing.

> —Autism and PDD Support Network,
> www.autism-pdd.net/autism-tips.html

100. Even if you don't agree with the methods that are being used, if your child is improving, recognize it.

> —Autism and PDD Support Network,
> www.autism-pdd.net/autism-tips.html

101. Maintain a "we" attitude. Ask how "we" can work together to solve a given problem.

> —Autism and PDD Support Network,
> www.autism-pdd.net/autism-tips.html

102. Write articles to the local paper about one of your child's success stories. It's good for the school, the teacher, and your child.

—Autism and PDD Support Network,
www.autism-pdd.net/autism-tips.html

103. If you're part of a parent group, consider inviting teachers and/ or administrators to a meeting every now and again. They are probably curious about what parent groups talk about and would appreciate being included in discussions. Their perspectives are often very enlightening, and they might have concerns that never occurred to the parents. Remember, inclusion isn't only for kids.

—Autism and PDD Support Network,
www.autism-pdd.net/autism-tips.html

104. Work on creating a good relationship with all the people who work with your child. Be open to sharing information about your child.

—Autism and PDD Support Network,
www.autism-pdd.net/autism-tips.html

105. Be willing to take part. Volunteer to help out. Be as involved as possible.

> —Autism and PDD Support Network,
> www.autism-pdd.net/autism-tips.html

106. Remember people at the end of each year. Little notes or gifts of thanks will be very appreciated by those who receive them.

> —Autism and PDD Support Network,
> www.autism-pdd.net/autism-tips.html

107. Document your child's condition and school requirements. If your child is diagnosed with an autism spectrum disorder, make sure that the school has a copy of the diagnosis. This might seem obvious, but in some cases the school and district have been able to point out that they were unaware of any actual diagnosis of autism disorder.

> —Harold L. Doherty, "Tips for Securing a Teachers Assistant
> for Your Autistic Student," www.wellsphere.com/autism-autism
> -spectrum-article/ta-tips-tips-for-securing-a-teachers-
> assistant-for-your-autistic-student/146550

108. One very effective way to keep communication open is to use logbooks. The teachers (and others who are working with your child) write in these each day and send them back home with the child. The parent reads what the teacher(s) write and responds and sends the book back with the child. These are especially effective with nonverbal children. It keeps the communication open between parent and teacher(s). Plus, sometimes writing to a teacher makes it easier to communicate an idea exactly the way you want to express it.

—Autism and PDD Support Network,
www.autism-pdd.net/autism-tips.html

109. Inform teachers immediately of any unusual circumstances occurring at home. A stressed child cannot attend to tasks, often exhibits disruptive behavior, or might simply space out. Teachers might misread these signs. Examples range from divorce to a sick grandmother to a new baby. Each student has a very different response to these life changes.

—Autism and PDD Support Network,
www.autism-pdd.net/autism-tips.html

110. Remember that working with the school can be a very emotional, personal process, because this is your child. It's very easy to feel defensive. Try to describe your needs in behavioral terms, not emotional terms.

> —Autism and PDD Support Network,
> www.autism-pdd.net/autism-tips.html

111. Keep things in perspective: Ask yourself, "Is what my child doing typical for his age group, or does his behavior have to do with his disability?" Encourage those who work with your child to do so, too.

> —Autism and PDD Support Network,
> www.autism-pdd.net/autism-tips.html

112. Know that everything you do is not written in stone. You can change things. Just because you decided something at the end of June doesn't mean you have to do it for the next year. You can change it at the end of October if it's not working. You can call the committee back and ask to reevaluate the situation.

> —Autism and PDD Support Network,
> www.autism-pdd.net/autism-tips.html

113. Remember to think of your child first. The disability is just part of who your child is. Remind people of your child's strengths. Encourage teachers to praise him.

> —Autism and PDD Support Network,
> www.autism-pdd.net/autism-tips.html

114. Ask the teacher to have your child be in the helper position at times, not always the one being helped.

> —Autism and PDD Support Network,
> www.autism-pdd.net/autism-tips.html

115. Ask that your child participate in everything, even at a modified level of activity.

> —Autism and PDD Support Network,
> www.autism-pdd.net/autism-tips.html

116. Make a list of things you want to say before you go to a meeting and take it with you. When you meet, give yourself plenty of time to discuss important issues.

> —Autism and PDD Support Network,
> www.autism-pdd.net/autism-tips.html

117. If you know an autism advocate or fellow parent of an autistic child who would be willing to attend a meeting with the school, you should bring them along. They can provide you with moral support and confirmation of your experiences as a parent in describing what your child requires.

—Harold L. Doherty, "Tips for Securing a Teachers Assistant for Your Autistic Student," www.wellsphere.com/autism-autism -spectrum-article/ta-tips-tips-for-securing-a-teachers- assistant-for-your-autistic-student/146550

118. If your child requires an individual-based learning method using Applied Behavior Analysis (ABA) techniques, or other individual- based instructions, emphasize this with the school. For ABA in particular there is a great deal of professional literature about the need for one-to-one instruction for autistic children.

—Harold L. Doherty, "Tips for Securing a Teachers Assistant for Your Autistic Student," www.wellsphere.com/autism-autism -spectrum-article/ta-tips-tips-for-securing-a-teachers- assistant-for-your-autistic-student/146550

CHAPTER 9

Adjusting to School

119. If the new school year involves getting up earlier than has been the case over the summer, it might be helpful to phase this in gradually, well before the start of school. It might also be useful to phase in the rhythm of mealtimes that will be in place during the school year.

—Lars Perner, PhD, www.AspergersSyndrome.org

120. If the child will be wearing different clothes to school than he did during vacation, it might be helpful to phase this in ahead of time as well.

—Lars Perner, PhD, www.AspergersSyndrome.org

121. If a new school, or a new room at the old school, is involved, it might be important to see it before the start of the term. The classroom should be examined for possible sensory violations (e.g., creaking doors, lights that might be flickering, fans that might be running in the background, echo, or unusual odors).

—Lars Perner, PhD, www.AspergersSyndrome.org

122. If information about the child's schedule for the coming year is available, it might be better to know this before the start of the year rather than on the first day. If new subjects start this year, advance notice of what these classes involve is essential, and it is important to look for potential problems.

—Lars Perner, PhD, www.AspergersSyndrome.org

123. Ensure that the school has a "home base" for your son on the spectrum if he is mainstreamed or fully included—a quiet and safe place where he can go to review information needed for his class, or to cope with any stresses and behavioral challenges.

124. If there is a new teacher, this will of course be a considerable adjustment. Obviously, it would be helpful to meet this teacher (with just the child and family present) before school starts. To get a sense of expectations, it would be useful to know this teacher's rules as explicitly as possible before school starts.

—Lars Perner, PhD, www.AspergersSyndrome.org

125. Individualized social "rule" cards can be taped to the child's desk as a visual reminder regarding appropriate social behaviors to exhibit. The rules can be written on index cards, illustrated, laminated, and then taped onto the desk.

—Roger Pierangelo and George A. Giuliani,
Teaching Students with Autism Spectrum Disorders

126. *If something is bothering me, I can . . .* This visual card can be taped to the child's desk or placed in a small photo album with the following illustrated examples:

- Raise my hand for help
- Close my eyes and count to ten
- Take five big breaths
- Ask for a break

—Roger Pierangelo and George A. Giuliani,
Teaching Students with Autism Spectrum Disorders

127. If a child is in a large class, learning new names and faces can be difficult. If photos are available, they might be helpful. If not, perhaps the teacher, parent, or aide might teach the child the name of one new student each day.

—Lars Perner, PhD, www.AspergersSyndrome.org

128. When I was a child, loud sounds like the school bell hurt my ears like a dentist drill hitting a nerve. Children with autism need to be protected from sounds that hurt their ears. The sounds that will cause the most problems are school bells, PA systems, buzzers on the scoreboard in the gym, and the sound of chairs scraping on the floor.

—Temple Grandin, PhD, author of *Thinking in Pictures* and
The Way I See It; www.autism.com/ind_teaching_tips.asp

129. The fear of a dreaded sound can cause bad behavior. If a child covers his ears, it is an indicator that a certain sound hurts his ears. Sometimes sound sensitivity to a particular sound, such as the fire alarm, can be desensitized by recording the sound on a tape recorder. This will allow the child to initiate the sound and gradually increase its volume. The child must have control of playback of the sound.

—Temple Grandin, PhD, author of *Thinking in Pictures* and
The Way I See It; www.autism.com/ind_teaching_tips.asp

130. Some children might need to be warned in advance about fire drills.

131. Children should be taught when they are at a low stress level. This ensures that the child will more focused during learning and also reduces the likelihood of the child having a meltdown over a secondary issue that is not related to learning.

132. Some autistic people are bothered by visual distractions and fluorescent lights. They can see the flicker of the sixty-cycle electricity. To avoid this problem, place the child's desk near the window or try to avoid using fluorescent lights. If the lights cannot be avoided, use the newest bulbs you can get. New bulbs flicker less. The flickering of fluorescent lights can also be reduced by putting a lamp with an old-fashioned incandescent lightbulb next to the child's desk.

> —Temple Grandin, PhD, author of *Thinking in Pictures* and *The Way I See It*; www.autism.com/ind_teaching_tips.asp

133. Some hyperactive autistic children who fidget all the time will often be calmer if they are given a padded weighted vest to wear. Pressure from the garment helps to calm the nervous system. I was greatly calmed by pressure. For best results, the vest should be worn for twenty minutes and then taken off for a few minutes. This prevents the nervous system from adapting to it.

—Temple Grandin, PhD, author of *Thinking in Pictures* and *The Way I See It*; www.autism.com/ind_teaching_tips.asp

134. Some nonverbal children and adults cannot process visual and auditory input at the same time. They are mono-channel. They cannot see and hear at the same time. They should not be asked to look and listen at the same time. They should be given either a visual task or an auditory task. Their immature nervous system is not able to process simultaneous visual and auditory input.

—Temple Grandin, PhD, author of *Thinking in Pictures* and *The Way I See It*; www.autism.com/ind_teaching_tips.asp

CHAPTER 10

Options for Homeschooling

135. Contact the Home School Legal Defense Association, their website will provide information about the laws in each state, which tend to vary as to subjects required and parent qualifications.

136. When designing your own curriculum check out homeschool support groups (google) and The World Book, which provides an online guide (for free) detailing typical courses for each grade.

The following tips are adapted from "Beginning to Homeschool a Child with an Autism Spectrum Disorder" by Valorie Delp, Families. com, http://homeschooling.families.com/blog/7-tips-for-beginning-to-homeschool-a-child-an-autism-spectrum-disorder.

137. Most experts seem to feel that the beginning of homeschooling for a child with an ASD is to "de-school." The technical definition of this would be for your child to "unlearn" all the negative socialization experiences he had in school. Many homeschooling veterans point to this as a time for you to observe your child, and for your child to really explore areas that interest him. Learning must again become fun.

138. While "de-schooling," contact local organizations and support groups. Try to make contact with other parents who understand both autism and homeschooling.

139. Keep a journal. You might want to consider taking notes at this time. What helps your child focus? What are his favorite things, and what is he doing when happiest? Where does he excel?

140. Read books beyond autism! Many people have cited this as a very helpful and important step. A few favorites are: 7 Kinds of Smart, The Way They Learn, Stumbling on Happiness, and The Mindbody Prescription.

141. Ditch your preconceptions. Try to approach the process with an open mind. Think about your end goal and then work backwards: What will get you to your end goal with your child? It is likely to look different than traditional schooling would be, and that's just fine!

142. Determine where your child is on checklists and evaluations. Set a goal and then work toward that goal. On the other hand . . . ditch the checklist if it is too frustrating. In states where there is a lot of paperwork, you can document your child's progress toward the goal and why you stopped pursuing it.

143. Locate needed therapies and services for your child. There is a variety of resources available, and with a little legwork at the library, I've heard of many parents providing needed therapy at home as appropriate.

144. There are software programs that teach skills in the areas of attention, language, and social interaction, and they are taught using effective behavioral methods. I don't recommend that Computer-Based Intervention (CBI) be implemented twenty-five hours a week, but I do feel that it needs to be an integral part of a home-based intervention program.

—Valerie Herskowitz, "Computer-Based Intervention—
What's It All About?," *Cutting-Edge Therapies for Autism*

145. When getting down to working with your son at home, create a quiet workspace without any distractions. Try to have this place dedicated to work so that your son knows it will be all business when he is in this particular place.

....

Therapy Implementation—Armed Struggle

B e open-minded when choosing among the various therapies; remember the proverb of the "empty cup":

> A learned man once went to visit a Zen teacher to inquire about Zen. As the Zen teacher talked, the learned man frequently interrupted to express his own opinion about this or that.
>
> Finally, the Zen teacher stopped talking and began to serve tea to the learned man. He poured the cup full, then kept pouring until the cup overflowed.
>
> "Stop," said the learned man. "The cup is full; no more can be poured in."
>
> "Like this cup, you are full of your own opinions," replied the Zen teacher. "If you do not first empty your cup, how can you taste my tea?"

CHAPTER 11

Paying for It All

146. Once your son is diagnosed as autistic, or anyplace on the spectrum, he is entitled to Medicaid. Google "Medicaid Waiver Programs" in your home state, and you will find organizations that will walk you through the application process, free of charge, and educate you as to just what benefits are included with the waiver programs.

147. When paying for medical expenses, utilize the bucket system:
- Bucket One: Insurance/Medicaid; if the expense is not covered, then use
- Bucket Two: Flexible Spending Accounts; if not eligible (or if they are already used up), then use
- Bucket Three: Medical Expense Deduction. If it can be deemed a "good medical expense," save it for tax season.

148. Know the name and address and phone number for the "commissioner of insurance" for your state. If any autism-related claim (that you think should be covered by your plan) is denied or delayed, or you are getting the runaround, tell the insurer verbally that you will be contacting "the named insurance commissioner." Follow up with them in writing via a fax that you are bringing this to your state's "commissioner of insurance," and they will usually pay you. Pronto! Nobody likes to be turned in to their boss when they are playing stall-tactic games!

—Nadine Chikuni

149. ABA, AVB, Floortime, speech, physical therapy, occupational therapy, listening therapy, and sensory integration therapy are often *not* covered by the health insurance that is deducted from your paycheck by your employer. When there is coverage, most private insurance policies have service limitations, out-of-pocket expenses, and lifetime caps.

—Lynn and Randy Gaston, *Three Times the Love*

150. Remember that insurance is a business—your provider wants to take in more money than it pays out. This is definitely an area in which the squeaky wheel gets the grease.

151. You may also find additional resources through state or local laws that are designed to help children with handicaps (which includes autism, but may not specify as such—for instance, handicapped parking). Research available services provided for your child in your immediate area to obtain maximum benefits, talk to parent "mavens," and ask your local state representatives; they are eager to help their constituents.

152. While you will likely need to rearrange your work schedule or even your career, keep in mind that one parent should keep a good insurance plan, either from an employer or through some association. Medical costs and therapies are very expensive and beyond most people's means without the aid of insurance. Also remember once your child has an official diagnosis they are entitled to Medicaid, which has some pros and cons and is covered throughout the book.

153. While there is some help from the government, most notable Medicaid, there is not nearly enough. Your child can qualify for Supplemental Security Income (SSI), but this and the Medicaid benefits will only go so far. You will have to drain savings and borrow from any possible deep pockets, especially if you pursue biomedical treatments, most of which are not covered by any insurance. Unfortunately for the best outcomes you will need an intensive (read: expensive) program and will have to make decisions that will not necessarily be sound from a financial perspective. Just remember that things will only get more expensive in the long run without progress so though it may seem you are acting in the short term to create an intensive program, in reality it will be beneficial in the long term.

CHAPTER 12

Military Families with a Child with an ASD
Provided by Lisa Rupe

154.
Keep your own copy of all of your child's medical records.

155.
Enroll your child in the Exceptional Family Member Program (EFMP) and Extended Care Health Option (ECHO) to receive Applied Behavior Analysis (ABA).

156.
Network with other parents through listservs and Web sites to research the services and schools when you have a permanent change of station (PCS).

157.
Review special education law every time you PCS. Document everything after you PCS so the new district cannot drag its feet in anticipation of you leaving again.

158.
Understand how to file claims with TRICARE and Express Scripts (see www.tacanow.org/resources/military-resources.htm). Many biomedical treatment options are covered by TRICARE.

159.
Ask if you can be placed higher on the waiting list for housing because you have a special-needs child enrolled in EFMP.

160. Military dependents are not required to be immunized unless they attend Department of Defense (DoD) schools or day-care centers. Learn about medical and administrative exemptions.

161. Try to use the same doctor every time you visit a Military Treatment Facility (MTF).

162. Supplements are covered if they are available at the MTF pharmacy or if they contain at least one prescription ingredient.

163. Respite services vary from branch to branch and even base to base. Find out from your EFMP coordinator what is available at your installation or from the community.

164. Speak up. Use your chain of command and chaplain if you have a problem.

165. Military parents of disabled children provide the best resources for each other. Check out Specialized Training of Military Parents (STOMP) and their list of parents around the world who offer training to other parents (see www.StompProject.org). Also visit American Military Families Autism Support (on Facebook) and www.AutismSalutes.com.

CHAPTER 13

How to Build a Treatment Team

166. Remember to develop relationships with the teachers, doctors, and therapists who work with your son. Share information often; consider yourself the "team" leader.

167. Communicate with all of the individuals who are part of the team educating your child. By developing a team atmosphere or approach and consistently using structured programs, your son will receive the best treatment possible. All individuals involved in this team structure need to work together to reach common goals.

168. Every member of the treatment team needs to agree on the program, goals, and treatment for the child. Open communication is also essential. This ensures that everyone is working together to achieve the same objectives, which provides consistency and reinforcement of the objectives.

169. Your child should always be happy to see his/her therapist. If not, reevaluate the program.

170. Document everything. You will continually call upon all of your autism documents, notes, and records. Organizing your documents will also improve communication between a multidisciplinary health team—not to mention reduce your stress levels!

171. Scan and make copies of printed forms and print any online forms in case you need them during phone calls and meetings.

172. A treatment program containing a greater number of therapies or therapists does not necessarily mean better treatment. Having a smaller number of treatment providers can allow for deeper relationships between child and therapists, and parents and therapists. The more therapists who work with your boy with ASD, the more likely [your child will be] fragmented.

—Lauren Tobing-Puente, PhD, Licensed Psychologist,
www.drtobingpuente.com

173. Trust your gut when seeking a new treatment provider. You should feel comfortable very early on with your son's therapists. Even those with the best reputations do not always mean the best fit for your son, you, and your family.

—Lauren Tobing-Puente, PhD, Licensed Psychologist, www.drtobingpuente.com

174. One measure of a therapist's effectiveness is your child's progress. Is your child experiencing success with this therapist? If not, why? Watch the way your child reacts to the therapist during a treatment session, and vice versa. Is your child happy [to be with the therapist]? Is the therapist happy [to be with your child]?

—Karen Siff Exkorn, *The Autism Sourcebook*

175. Stay actively involved in your child's treatment. Sit in on some of your child's therapy sessions. Ask questions. Listen to your therapists' feedback. Learn how to reinforce some of the skills that your child is being taught. Offer your own feedback.

—Karen Siff Exkorn, *The Autism Sourcebook*

176. Learn about the different therapies being used on your son. Keep in mind that a certain therapy might not work for your child. Remember that the definition of insanity is doing the same old thing and expecting different results, so don't be afraid to consider other options.

CHAPTER 14

Applied Behavior Analysis (ABA) Therapy

177. Applied Behavior Analysis (ABA) therapy is a treatment model that is extremely effective in remediating many of the cognitive-, attention-, and language-based areas of deficit typical to autism. ABA is currently one of the most common interventions, and the core of many educational programs for treating children on the autism spectrum.

—Jenifer Clark, MA, PhD (c), "Applied Behavior Analysis,"
Cutting-Edge Therapies for Autism

178. Applied Behavior Analysis (ABA) is an empirically supported methodology that effectively teaches critical skills to children with autism. An ABA program will typically focus on communication skills, social skills, fine and gross motor skills, and cognitive skills. The basic principles of reinforcement are used to motivate the otherwise unmotivated learner. As the child becomes more connected socially to others, primary reinforcements (such as food) can be replaced by social reinforcers such as praise and tickles. The goals that are set for each child are broken down into their component parts so that the child will be successful. Problem behaviors are either extinguished or replaced. These undesired behaviors can be replaced with alternative behaviors that compete with the unwanted behavior. The positive behavior is heavily reinforced until it replaces the negative behavior so that it is more likely to occur in a given situation.

—Jenifer Clark, MA, PhD (c), MERIT Consulting

179. ABA treatment should begin as early as possible. Children who receive more treatment hours per week (i.e., thirty or more) have better outcomes than those who receive fewer (e.g., fifteen or less); continuing ABA treatment for two or more years will lead to the optimal outcome.

> —Dr. Doreen Granpeesheh, Dr. Jonathan Tarbox, and Dr. Michele Bishop, "Center for Autism and Related Disorders, Inc. (CARD)," *Cutting-Edge Therapies for Autism*

180. Children with ASD might not acquire skills through daily interactions in their home or school environment. To effectively teach children with ASD, tasks are broken down into small, measurable units, and each skill is practiced repeatedly until the child masters the skill. Some skills might serve as building blocks for other more-complex skills (e.g., imitation, attending). Thus, we might begin working on more-basic skills that allow children to acquire building blocks that prepare the child to learn more advanced skills and learn in a number of different environments. Once a skill is mastered, it is practiced periodically to make sure the child continues to maintain previously mastered skills over time.

> —Dr. Tiffany Kodak and Dr. Alison Betz, "Center for Autism Spectrum Disorders, Munroe-Meyer Institute," *Cutting-Edge Therapies for Autism*

181. Some children might find imitating actions challenging because of their difficulty attending to the visual information being presented. A child with these particular issues would be best served by an intervention that drew their attention to the visual demonstration (perhaps waiting until the child is looking, or attracting their visual attention prior to engaging in the action). Other children might have difficulty translating what they have observed into a message that allows them to imitate the movement.

—Jenifer Clark, MA, PhD (c), "Applied Behavior Analysis,"
Cutting-Edge Therapies for Autism

182. The more that parents of children with autism can incorporate sound behavioral practices in a natural way with their autistic child, the better that child's prognosis will be.

—Jenifer Clark, MA, PhD (c), "Applied Behavior Analysis,"
Cutting-Edge Therapies for Autism

183. Many children with autism quickly come to appreciate social interactions as powerful reinforcers but it may take some specific interventions early on in the treatment to allow them to benefit from these more typical interactions.

—Jenifer Clark, MA, PhD (c), "Applied Behavior Analysis,"
Cutting-Edge Therapies for Autism

CHAPTER 15

Behavioral Treatment Plans

The following tips are from Steve Kossor;
www.TreatmentPlansThatWorked.com

184. A behavioral treatment plan should provide all of the information necessary for a conscientious person to deliver the correct treatment procedures, at the correct times, and with sufficient consistency to produce the changes in behavior that are described in the plan—reducing or eliminating undesirable behavior and increasing or improving desired behavior, while providing a means to monitor progress on an ongoing basis that informs the process of treatment.

185. Any behavioral treatment plan should specify the *exact* behavior that is "targeted" for improvement. The plan must say *exactly* what is to be reduced or eliminated. By the same token, the plan must say *exactly* what is to be taught in replacement of the "targeted" behavior. It is rarely helpful to tell a child what *not* to do; you always have to specify what he *should do* as well.

186. A treatment plan should explain *exactly* what the treatment provider should be doing to accomplish the replacement of the "target" behavior. A treatment provider should be able to look at the treatment plan and know precisely which techniques are to be used, how often, and in which circumstances. When terms like "contingency contracting" are used, a glossary of terms that is accessible to the treatment provider is *essential*. How else can the treatment provider know *exactly* what to do?

187. A treatment plan should always contain a simple and easy means of measuring progress from the perspective of the treatment *recipient*, not the treatment provider. Outcome progress measurement should include a "baseline" measure, which is a starting point in the measurement of treatment outcomes that precedes the start of the treatment period. How else will you know how far you've come (or how far you've gone astray) if you don't know where you started?

188. Treatment plans must include a planned stop date, so that the treatment team can prepare to present information to funding authorities prior to that date in order for funding to be continued. Continued funding is necessary and therefore justifiable whenever the child is within the age served by the funding entity, the treatment plan is *working*, but the work has not yet been satisfactorily completed.

CHAPTER 16

Developmental and Relationship Therapies

189. Floortime: Play with a Purpose. For many kids the most challenging deficits are social and communication delays. These can be addressed through fun parent–child engagements known as Floortime. I recommend parents read *Engaging Autism* by Stanley Greenspan and give it a try. Learn more about Floortime at the link below, there are instructional videos, information on therapies and how to get trained yourself: www.icdl.com/dirFloortime/overview/index.shtml.

190. Other therapies parents can do themselves include Relationship Development Intervention (RDI) and the Son-Rise program. You will need to be trained by certified consultants in each, but can then implement the programs at home. Check out www.RDIconnect.com and www.AutismTreatmentCenter.org for more information and therapists in your area.

191. Parents are taught to increase their experience sharing language and decrease their instrumental language. By providing the child with ASD language that does not require a specific response, parents are teaching the child the true value of language: to share with others.

—Laura Hynes, "Relationship Development Intervention," *Cutting-Edge Therapies for Autism*

192. Improvement is likely, recovery is possible! There are too many kids who have improved and outright recovered for you to dismiss these outcomes. Work is required yes, and frankly, many may not be up to the task. But if you keep in mind that all is possible, you will be better able to maintain momentum. Just remember that these kids have the capacity to improve; meet them halfway!

193. Join in their world. If you take the approach pioneered by Stanley Greenspan, you can engage the child by entering their world. Join in their stim or playfully obstruct it in order to engage the child. An example would be to physically block an item or location they want to go. My son likes to tap a certain area on the floor. If I sit there, he needs to get me to move, which requires some level of effort and communication. Think of it as turning into a skid on a slick road in order to gain control of the car.

194. Tasks should be fun. Though it is work to teach your child, the more fun you (and your child's therapists) make it the greater engagement and motivation you will receive from your child.

195. Make the child feel comfortable. They may not appear to be paying attention to you, but the will sense your disposition, make it positive and welcoming. Use high affect and positivity to engage the child.

196. Remember your son cannot go from zero to sixty then back down to zero. A typical child can learn to step back and take a breath, but a child with autism can spin himself into his own world, you need to go in and bring him out.

CHAPTER 17

Physical/Occupational Therapy

197. The earliest forms of physical therapy might include working on skills such as sitting, rolling, crawling, standing, and walking. As the children get older, they might receive physical therapy to address concerns regarding muscle strength, endurance, balance, coordination, motor planning, ball skills, and various forms of locomotion.

—Meghan Collins, "Physical Therapy,"
Cutting-Edge Therapies for Autism

198. Educational concepts can be embedded into physical activities utilizing equipment that meets students' different sensory profiles, and students can experience learning in a way that empowers them and gives them an outlet for their individual learning styles.

—Amanda Friedman and Alison Berkley,
"Sensory Gym: Emerge and See," *Cutting-Edge Therapies for Autism*

199. Find an occupational therapist: Many children with ASD and sensory integration dysfunction present with low muscle tone and a tendency to rely on end ranges of their joints for stability. This can be illustrated by a child who toe-walks with his back arched, chest out, and his shoulders back. Another example of this is a child who "W"-sits with a rounded back, shoulders forward, and head and neck tilted up. These postures can prevent components of typical movement from occurring that interfere with a child's ability to interact with their world. Both postures prevent side-to-side weight shifting and, in turn, rotation of the trunk. Without rotation, a child's ability to integrate visual, auditory, movement, and spatial information might be significantly impacted.

—Markus Jarrow, "The SMILE Center,"
Cutting-Edge Therapies for Autism

200. Check out occupational therapy—a form of therapy designed to address both sensory needs and motor planning which virtually all ASD kids have. Therapists use a wide variety of tools, including balls, manipulatives, and even Play-Doh to help children learn to tolerate noises, textures, and certain environments. It's also used to address both fine and gross motor skills.

201. Occupational therapists can provide valuable insight, both practical and neurological, to help families better understand many of the questions they struggle with when raising a child with an autism spectrum disorder. Occupational therapy and sensory integration (SI) can be very effective treatment approaches for children with ASD.

> —Markus Jarrow, "Occupational Therapy and Sensory Integration," *Cutting-Edge Therapies for Autism*

202. A child who relies on self-stimulatory or self-regulatory behaviors to control their arousal level, or tune out adverse stimuli, is a child less available for engagement, learning, and skill acquisition.

> —Markus Jarrow, "Occupational Therapy and Sensory Integration," *Cutting-Edge Therapies for Autism*

203. No matter how effective the clinician is, he or she might only have an hour or two a week with the child. It is therefore essential that a home program be implemented. This might include simple modifications to the home, adaptations to the child's routines, toys, clothing, etc., as well as specific, scheduled treatment strategies to be carried out in the home and/or school. This is referred to as a sensory diet. This piece is critical in ensuring optimal progress.

> —Markus Jarrow, "Occupational Therapy and Sensory Integration," *Cutting-Edge Therapies for Autism*

204. Sensory issues can often be mistaken for behavioral problems. If a child has vestibular and visual issues, which impact his perception of his position in space, he might have great difficulty sitting upright in a chair without falling from time to time. To avoid falls or embarrassment, he might fidget to better process his body, or get out of his seat often. He, in turn, will present as a child who "won't" stay seated.

—Markus Jarrow, "Occupational Therapy and Sensory Integration," *Cutting-Edge Therapies for Autism*

205. With children with sensory integration dysfunction, it is important to remember that these behaviors might be nothing more than effective coping mechanisms. When the underlying sensory issues are addressed, the behavior might disappear altogether.

—Markus Jarrow, "Occupational Therapy and Sensory Integration," *Cutting-Edge Therapies for Autism*

206. Children inherently attempt to provide themselves with what they need and avoid what they are frightened by. They constantly listen to their bodies and try to regulate themselves. By listening to what their bodies tell us, we can help them to make a great deal of positive change.

—Markus Jarrow, "Occupational Therapy and Sensory Integration," *Cutting-Edge Therapies for Autism*

207. Play is an open doorway into engaging with students with ASD and the start of a teaching relationship with them.

—Amanda Friedman and Alison Berkley, "Sensory Gym: Emerge and See," *Cutting-Edge Therapies for Autism*

208. There are two main types of sensory play most children crave: manipulation of self and objects, and release of emotion and energy.

—Amanda Friedman and Alison Berkley, "Sensory Gym: Emerge and See," *Cutting-Edge Therapies for Autism*

209. Students thrive when learning is interwoven with physical release.

—Amanda Friedman and Alison Berkley, "Sensory Gym: Emerge and See," *Cutting-Edge Therapies for Autism*

210. We must begin to cater to students not only for their fundamental deficits, but to amplify their ever-present, yet often splintered *abilities* as well. Challenging students to reach their maximum success is not defined by our standard views of education, but rather, what they need to function within their families and communities. Teaching students within a sensory gym setting lends itself to great joy, trust between teacher and student, and generalization with peers and activities found outside a typical classroom.

—Amanda Friedman and Alison Berkley, "Sensory Gym: Emerge and See," *Cutting-Edge Therapies for Autism*

211. Limited range of motion or muscle flexibility might be addressed by traditional stretching or massage.

—Meghan Collins, "Physical Therapy," *Cutting-Edge Therapies for Autism*

212. Aerobic fitness might be a concern, as weight gain and lethargy are common side effects of various medications children on the autism spectrum might take. Traditional exercise might be performed during therapy sessions, such as push-ups, sit-ups, or jumping jacks, to improve aerobic capacity.

—Meghan Collins, "Physical Therapy," *Cutting-Edge Therapies for Autism*

213. Balance activities might include negotiating stairs with and without support from the railing or wall, walking across a balance beam, standing on one foot, hopping, moving onto, off of, or across uneven or movable surfaces, and roller-skating.

—Meghan Collins, "Physical Therapy,"
Cutting-Edge Therapies for Autism

214. If a child is having difficulty catching a medium-size ball, balloons serve as good substitutes until the child becomes more familiar with the task.

—Meghan Collins, "Physical Therapy,"
Cutting-Edge Therapies for Autism

215. A child receiving physical therapy will improve their gross motor function, which is an important aspect of socialization, allowing the child to participate in general play, physical education, or sports. The key to a successful physical therapy session is making the activities during the session motivating for the child. Ultimately kids just want to have fun!

—Meghan Collins, "Physical Therapy,"
Cutting-Edge Therapies for Autism

CHAPTER 18

Vision Therapy

216.

Does he need vision therapy? We ask questions like: Do both eyes perceive the same image at the same time? Do both eyes move in unison? Do both eyes have equal focusing power? Do both eyes do all these visual requirements easily, fluidly, and for an extended length of time? If the answer to any of these questions is "No," then vision therapy might be indicated.

—Dr. Jeffrey Becker, "Vision Therapy,"
Cutting-Edge Therapies for Autism

The following checklist is excerpted from the chapter "Vision Therapy" by Dr. Jeffrey Becker in *Cutting-Edge Therapies for Autism*.

If you can answer yes to two or more of these signs, your child should engage in a complete neurosensory and developmental vision evaluation:

- Child likes to look out of the corners of his eyes when doing either near point or distance viewing.
- Child only does near tasks for short periods of time, then goes back to task after a few short minutes.
- Child turns head to the left or right to view distant or near objects.
- Child bends head to either shoulder when viewing distant or near objects.
- Child covers or closes an eye when looking at near point tasks.

- Child likes to visually stim with his hands in front of one eye or another.
- Child moves closer and closer to near point tasks over a short period of time.
- Child rubs eyes frequently.
- Child's eyes tend to water when doing near point tasks.
- Child likes to turn head up or down and moves head in strange positions to do near point tasks.

---

217. Fifty-three percent of children who are poor readers have some form of visual functioning disorder, and it has been estimated that up to 80 percent of children with special needs have significant visual functioning disorders that affect the learning and developmental process.

—Dr. Jeffrey Becker, "Vision Therapy,"
Cutting-Edge Therapies for Autism

218. Vision therapy can be done in an office by a trained therapist, in an outpatient rehabilitation center, or at home. Vision rehabilitation to correct most oculomotor, eye-focusing, and eye-deviation deficits typically continues for six to eight months when done two or three times per week. Treatment also requires home participation for thirty to forty-five minutes per day for five days per week on an outpatient basis. This does not mean that the rehabilitation cannot be concluded earlier (or later) than this prescribed time. Program length is dependent on the child's participation level and attendance.

—Dr. Jeffrey Becker, "Vision Therapy,"
Cutting-Edge Therapies for Autism

219. Children and adults who fear escalators often have visual processing problems. They fear the escalator because they cannot determine when to get on or off. These individuals might also not be able to tolerate fluorescent lights. The Irlen colored glasses might be helpful for them.

—Temple Grandin, PhD, author of *Thinking in Pictures* and *The Way I See It*; www.autism.com/ind_teaching_tips.asp

CHAPTER 19
Speech-Language Therapy

220. Take your child for an evaluation by a speech-language pathologist (SLP), as he will likely need speech therapy.

221. Speech-Language Therapy can provide remediation for the following communication disorders:

- Language disorder: impairment of receptive (comprehension), expressive (use of spoken), written, and/or other symbol systems;
- Speech disorder: impairment of the articulation of speech sounds, fluency or voice;
- Pragmatic disorder: impairment of the ability to use and understand social language (verbal and nonverbal);
- Hearing disorder: impairment of the auditory system;
- Central auditory processing disorder: impairment of the ability to process, retrieve, and/or organize information through the peripheral and central nervous systems;
- Prosody disorder: impairment of the suprasegmentals of speech (intonation, stress).

—Lavina Pereira and Michelle Solomon,
"Speech-Language Therapy," *Cutting-Edge Therapies for Autism*

222. Children ages zero to three and school-age children might be eligible for speech and language services through the state in which they reside. Government agencies within your state will be able to provide contact information to begin the assessment process, which will determine eligibility for services. School-age children might be evaluated to determine the need for speech-language therapy within the school setting. In addition, licensed therapists in your area can be located by visiting the American Speech-Language-Hearing Association (ASHA) website (www.ASHA.org), asking your child's doctor, or by contacting local support groups and agencies.

—Lavina Pereira and Michelle Solomon,
"Speech-Language Therapy," *Cutting-Edge Therapies for Autism*

223. When working with a child on the autism spectrum, it is vital that the surroundings are modified to lessen distractions and provide support for additional needs, such as sensory and attention deficits.

- Decrease visual distractions (little or no decorations)
- Supportive seating
- Facing away from the window
- Good lighting
- Established work area and sensory or "break" area
- Awareness of noises that might be distracting to the child (buzzing of light, air conditioner, heat)
- Toys and materials out of reach and in enclosed cabinets

—Lavina Pereira and Michelle Solomon,
"Speech-Language Therapy," *Cutting-Edge Therapies for Autism*

224. These activities foster the development of early sight-reading and literacy:

- Use of pictures/words to create a daily schedule
- Use of pictures/words to create an activity schedule for one session to assist in transitioning from one activity to the next
- Written words on objects around room
- Choice board with pictures/words
- Use start-to-finish activities that have a clear beginning and end

—Lavina Pereira and Michelle Solomon,
"Speech-Language Therapy," *Cutting-Edge Therapies for Autism*

225.

These activities support and encourage communication and interaction:

- Use of routines (daily living activities—dressing, snack time, bedtime routine)
- Use of scripts to learn and practice social scenarios (inviting a peer to play)
- Social stories (address problematic situations by reading stories)
- Repetition of material to foster learning (books, songs, carrier phrases such as "I want _____")
- Use of cloze sentences ("Birds fly in the (sky)") and fill-ins ("Ready set (go)")
- "Sabotaging" of materials and environment (desired toy out of reach, piece of a toy missing)
- Group therapy (sessions with typical peers to provide modeling of appropriate social behavior)
- Sessions in a natural setting to promote carryover
- Use of technology (computers, handheld game systems) to encourage independent learning and visual feedback
- Establishing a routine to the sessions
- Keep pace of sessions relative to attention span

> —Lavina Pereira and Michelle Solomon,
> "Speech-Language Therapy," *Cutting-Edge Therapies for Autism*

226. A naturalistic setting promotes inclusion in "normal" everyday situations, teaches the individual how to interact with others, and allows for more "teachable" moments. Furthermore, when therapy is provided in a natural setting, activities are more purposeful and meaningful, which will increase your child's motivation and desire to participate. For example, an SLP would make learning the labels of food more salient if it is taught and experienced in a kitchen with real food items and engaging activities (cooking, cutting, tasting) versus through the use of pictures and pretend play food in an office or bedroom setting.

—Lavina Pereira and Michelle Solomon,
"Speech-Language Therapy," *Cutting-Edge Therapies for Autism*

227. Putting scratch-and-sniff and Braille on the Picture Exchange Communication System (PECS) is just a way to open up an avenue of communication for some of the kids who are severely impacted by their sensory processing problems. I first came up with the idea with a teen with no receptive or expressive language, who did not use PECS (except to hand them to us without looking at them until he got what he wanted), and did not respond to sign either. He did, however, sniff all his teachers, apparently to identify us. I've also used tactile sign (sign for the deaf/blind) with some of the kids. I tend to save these things for the "last-ditch" measure of desperation; for example, if a child is six and not responding to any of the standards of "Total Communication." I just try to make it a bit more "total" by addressing more senses. I haven't gotten to the last extreme yet, although if I run into someone who only tastes everything by the age of seven, I'll darn well glue lollipops (all-natural, gluten-free/casein-free) to his PECS to try to get SOMETHING through.

—Tara Marshall

CHAPTER 20

Music Therapy

228. Many children with autism enjoy and excel in musical activities. Parents can sing with their child, engage in movement and dance, and provide a box of toy instruments. Children with autism who develop an interest in an actual musical instrument can practice their lessons with a parent's encouragement.

> —Angie Geisler, "Fun Activity Suggestions for Parents of Children with Autism," www.brighthub.com/education /special/articles/57559.aspx#ixzz0l0QC6jNt

229. Music therapy is the clinical and evidence-based use of music interventions to accomplish individualized goals within a therapeutic relationship by a credentialed professional who has completed an approved music therapy program. It is a well-established allied health profession that uses music therapeutically to address behavioral, social, psychological, communicative, physical, sensory-motor, and/or cognitive functioning. Music therapists are members of an interdisciplinary team of education or health-care professionals who work collaboratively to address an individual's needs. For individuals with diagnoses on the autism spectrum, music therapy provides a unique variety of music experiences in a developmentally appropriate manner to effect changes in behavior and facilitate development of skills.

> —The American Music Therapy Association

230. The music that seems to work best for my autistic student is music he has heard before in video games or movies, famous tunes such as "Ode to Joy" and "Yankee Doodle," and very dramatic melodies, such as the first phrase from *Bach's Toccata in Dm*.

—Dana Thynes, www.Music-for-Music-Teachers.com/autism.html

231. I teach it the first time the way I want him to play it eventually; no simplified versions along the way to getting to the difficult version. His memory is too long, and apparently too inflexible.

—Dana Thynes, www.Music-for-Music-Teachers.com/autism.html

The following tips are adapted from the chapter "Music Therapy" by The American Music Therapy Association in *Cutting-Edge Therapies for Autism*. For more information visit www.musictherapy.org or call 310-589-3300.

232. How to find a board-certified music therapist: Some music therapists work in school settings as a related service on a child's IEP, either hired or contracted by a school district. Others have private practices or work for agencies that specialize in treatment for individuals with developmental disabilities.

233. Some states fund music therapy services through Medicaid waivers or other state programs.

---

234. Private health insurance reimbursement usually requires preapproval on a case-by-case basis.

235. Music therapy is a related service under IDEA and can be included on IEPs if deemed a necessary part of a child's special education program.

236. Music therapy offers a particularly important intervention for individuals with autism spectrum disorders to engage and foster their capacity for flexibility, creativity, variability, and tolerance of change. These interventions tend to balance the more structured and behaviorally driven education required in school settings.

237. Research has shown that people with diagnoses on the autism spectrum often show a heightened interest and response to music, making it an excellent therapeutic tool.

238. Because music is motivating and engaging, it may be used as a natural "reinforcer" for desired responses.

239. By the same token, some individuals with autism may not indicate an interest in music, or may seem to have an aversion to music because of sensory issues or because of unfamiliar settings, people, or activities. Music therapy can assist these individuals to gradually adapt to new situations and cope with sound sensitivities or individual differences in auditory processing.

240. The flexible nature of music therapy allows it to blend in with different theoretical approaches and models, so music therapists can work cooperatively with teams in various settings under a variety of treatment philosophies.

CHAPTER 21

Therapy Animals

241. The use of animals for the purpose of purportedly providing therapeutic benefit to humans has existed in the literature for several decades. Commonly known as pet therapy or pet care, outcomes reportedly include improvements related to self-confidence, receptive and expressive language skills, socialization, and problem-solving skills.

—Richard L. Simpson, *Autism Spectrum Disorders*

242. Some children will benefit hugely from a service dog—for others, the sensory stimulation will be overwhelming.

243. Consider a therapy pet. Pets, especially trained autism service dogs, are a wonderful help for children who wander away from home or for those who have difficulty in public situations.

—Bryna Siegel, *Helping Children with Autism Learn*

244. Service dogs must be worked as service dogs and not allowed to become family pets, and this, at times, can be difficult for other family members to understand or endorse. Parents must consistently use the service dog to interrupt their child's inappropriate behavior. Service dogs will quit working in as few as three weeks if their skills are not used adequately. At first this can be overwhelming for parents who are already stretched and exhausted. However, when parents succeed in their efforts, we see miracles occur with these children.

—Tiffany Denver, "Personal Service Canines,"
Cutting-Edge Therapies for Autism

245. Animals act as a social lubricant and ease the stress of therapy by being comforting. The animals also act as a link in conversation between clinician and client, helping to establish trust and rapport between patient and clinician. The mere presence of an animal can also give clients a sense of comfort, which further promotes rapport in the therapeutic relationship.

—Dr. Aubrey Fine, "Animal-Assisted Interventions and Persons with Autism Spectrum Disorders," *Cutting-Edge Therapies for Autism*

246. Children and adults with ASD might relate better with companion animals because they both use sensory-based thinking.

247. Sensory oversensitivity might have a tremendous impact on the outcome and is extremely variable. This means that some people might not be able to tolerate smells or sudden sounds from an animal. On the other hand, some will have no sensory problems with animals and will be attracted to them.

248. Animals, specifically dogs, might communicate their behavioral intentions more easily to persons with ASD, especially because their relationships are simpler.

249. The love and unconditional regard received from a pet or from a therapy animal might represent a catalyst for emotional and psychological growth.

—Dr. Aubrey Fine, "Animal-Assisted Interventions and
Persons with Autism Spectrum Disorders,"
Cutting-Edge Therapies for Autism

250. Recreational horseback riding therapy and licensed-therapist-directed hippotherapy are individually efficacious, and are both medically indicated as therapy for gross motor rehabilitation.

—Franklin Levinson and Dr. Nicola Start,
"Equine Therapy," *Cutting-Edge Therapies for Autism*

251. Hippotherapy has been shown to increase verbal communication skills in some autistic children in as little as eighteen to twenty-five minutes of riding once a week for eight weeks. "We see their arousal and affect change. They become more responsive to cues."

—Dr. Lewis Mehl-Madrona,
"Traditional and Indigenous Healing," *Cutting-Edge Therapies for Autism,*

252. The child can experience the power of the body of the horse as it moves and is given an enhanced sense of his or her own body, and thus, his or her sense of "self."

—Franklin Levinson and Dr. Nicola Start,
"Equine Therapy," *Cutting-Edge Therapies for Autism*

253. It is easier for children to learn empathy with animals because children view them as peers.

—Franklin Levinson and Dr. Nicola Start,
"Equine Therapy," *Cutting-Edge Therapies for Autism*

254. It has been clinically documented that just being around horses changes humans' brain-wave patterns. When we are with horses, we tend to calm down and become more focused. It is, therefore, no wonder that interaction with horses should prove therapeutic to grown-ups and children alike.

—Franklin Levinson and Dr. Nicola Start,
"Equine Therapy," *Cutting-Edge Therapies for Autism*

CHAPTER 22

Aquatic Therapy

Adapted from the chapter "Aquatic Therapy" by Andrea Salzman in *Cutting-Edge Therapies for Autism*. Visit www.aquatic-university.com for more information.

255. Benefits of aquatic therapy are many. Clinicians have reported a substantial increase in swim skills, attention, muscle strength, balance, tolerating touch, initiating/ maintaining eye contact, and water safety during their sessions with young children with autism.

256. In addition to the normal therapy pursuits of strengthening, balance training, and range of motion (ROM), the pool is an excellent location to work on:
- Transitional stress
- Social interactions
- Body awareness and kinesthesia
- Tactile processing
- Vestibular processing
- Visual processing

257. Water activities can provide autistic children with the opportunity to embrace change. Even the act of entering the pool from the deck is a massive leap into uncertainty, and parents looking for ways to promote acceptance of change can use the pool for this end.

258. As a shield, children often seek out a comfort place in the pool—a place where they feel the safest. Parents or therapists who choose to work in the water should work from the child's chosen safe spot, leave for a little bit, and return again and again.

259. Simple childhood games like whirlpool (running in one direction in a circle and then quickly reversing direction to move against the "current") can create opportunities for feedback loops which are unachievable on land.

260. The game "Simon says" can be used to both assess and encourage proprioceptive awareness. Make use of this kid's game to teach better body control. Or make use of wet, clingy items such as towels, fabric shower curtains, and even discarded clothing to morph a dress-up game into a therapeutic session designed to enhance proprioception.

261. It is possible to increase—or decrease—the amount of tactile input the child receives by putting him into the pool. But what if the child is so averse to noxious stimulation that he won't even place his face near the water's surface? Stock up a therapeutic toolbox with everyday items easily purchased, such as car-wash mitts, sponges, and window clings. In the water, it becomes possible to stroke cheeks with cheap paint rollers and drape soaking-wet bath towels over heads to increase tolerance for abrasive touch and pressure.

262. An inexpensive way to convert your therapy pool into a vestibular challenge is to perform hammock swings. Purchase a child's parachute or a net hammock. Spread out the parachute or hammock and have the child climb aboard. Swing the fabric through the water: up, down, side to side, tilted, and rotated. Move the child rapidly, then slowly, then rapidly again. The child can sit, kneel, lie supine, or even stand in the hammock during this task. To make this task more interactive, ask the child to sing in time to movements and to anticipate movements before they happen.

CHAPTER 23

Dance and Movement Therapy

The following tips are adapted from the chapter "Dance/Movement Therapy" by Mariah Meyer LeFeber in *Cutting-Edge Therapies for Autism*.

263. In application, dance/movement therapy fosters socialization and communication in clients who otherwise might find it difficult to relate. The ability to engage fully through nonverbal activity sets dance/movement therapy apart from other forms of therapy. It creates an affirming environment for clients, where they are able to experience the value of belonging. Ultimately, dance/movement therapy provides both a bridge for contact and a medium for reciprocal communication for children with autism.

264. When building treatment goals, each child with autism presents with specific needs and challenges, yet a handful of goals are generally applicable. The first of these goals is increasing sensory motor and perceptual motor development, directly targeting the motor deficits often faced by children with autism spectrum disorder. By working from both a functional and expressive standpoint, dance/movement therapists can use simple vocabulary and movement to stimulate perceptual, gross, and fine motor skills. An example of this is teaching children the perceptual concept of "in and out" by having them physically step inside of a space (i.e., a hula hoop) and then outside of that same space. Through the gross motor movement, the children experientially learn the concept, which can then be generalized to other areas.

117

265. Building off of the growing understanding of self vs. others, dance/movement therapy works to foster body awareness and nurture a client's personal self-concept. By reflecting a child's movement nonverbally and then translating what is seen into simple language (i.e., mirroring the child in moving their head side to side, while verbalizing "I see you moving your head"), the dance/movement therapist positively verbalizes how the child appears, inherently improving his body awareness or body image. The simple verbalizations, or the "noticing" of what is going on, also help to structure the experience for the participant (Loman, 1995). As an added benefit, this verbalization of action naturally increases the movement repertoire of the client (applicable to goal one), as he is exposed to not only the conscious experience of his own movement, but also that of the others in the room.

266. Since autism possibly relates to deficiencies in the mirror neuron system of the brain, dance/movement therapy has the potential to unlock and develop some of these deficient areas through the process of movement.

267. The American Dance Therapy Association (ADTA) is the professional organization for dance/movement therapists in the U.S. and beyond. To learn more about the field or find a dance/movement therapist in your area, visit their website at www.ADTA.org, or contact the national office by phone at (410) 997-4040.

CHAPTER 24

Art Therapy

The following tips are adapted from the chapter "Art Therapy Approaches to Treating Autism" by Nicole Martin and Dr. Donna Betts in *Cutting-Edge Therapies for Autism*.

268. Art projects designed to tackle specific treatment goals are limitless and may include group murals (to work on collaboration, reciprocity, and flexibility skills), portrait drawing (to work on face processing and relationship skills), friendship boxes (to work on memory and relationship skills), and many more.

269. A child on a gluten-free diet should avoid traditional play dough since it contains wheat flour.

270. It is especially important to offer a safe, predictable, and stable environment by providing therapy at the same time every week and setting up materials in an orderly fashion. By doing so, the art therapist establishes psychological continuity and a stable environment for the client.

271. Goals that a child with ASD might accomplish in art therapy include age-appropriate drawing or modeling skills, improved self-expression and reduced anxiety or frustration, independent or semi-independent use of art making as a coping skill or self-soothing tool, improved social skills such as project collaboration and flexibility, and age-appropriate imagination and ideation skills.

272. Art therapy has the potential to benefit the majority of individuals with autism, not just those who demonstrate a precocious talent.

273. Dr. Betts once worked with a student who was obsessed with his own wet saliva. The boy was fascinated with the patterns of movement he created with his spit, and this is what kept him engaged in the kinesthetic activity. Thus, Dr. Betts came up with a way to divert the boy away from his excessive interest in saliva by introducing a dry substance—sand. In his art therapy sessions, the boy was encouraged to play with sand and its containers in a tabletop box. As he learned about how to manipulate his environment through sand play, his obsession with the spit eventually disappeared. With Dr. Betts's continuous encouragement and praise for using the sand, contained within the boundaries of a box, the client progressed toward a more flexible and mature ego functioning.

274. Including art therapy as a component of early intervention treatment helps individuals with autism form good habits for a lifetime of using art as a vital means of expression.

SECTION 5

....

Medical and Nutritional Treatment

For many parents, working through the various biomedical treatments and associated diets are the most challenging components of the battle. It's easy to become overwhelmed with so much information. It's best to focus on one day and one treatment at a time, and remember—no matter how difficult the day, keep on breathing, because tomorrow is another day. The sun will rise, and who knows what Providence will bring.

CHAPTER 25

How to Find and Choose Your Doctors

275. Here are some questions to ask when choosing a doctor for your child:

- Approximately how many individuals with autism have you treated? What age range?

- In the event we have a biomedical-related emergency, how will I contact you?

- Do you share an e-mail address, cell-phone number, etc. with your patients?

- Can you collaborate with other specialists we will be dealing with (gastrointestinal, etc.)? Are you willing to collaborate on treatment and testing with my child's pediatrician if he or she is receptive?

- Will you provide a clear plan for supplements and where to purchase them?

- What are the primary medical specialties in which you were originally trained (i.e., pediatrics, family medicine)? What is now the primary focus of your practice? If you are not an MD or DO, in what field(s) are you licensed?

- Do you sell proprietary nutritional supplements or have a sales agreement with supplement suppliers? Do you sell supplements at cost?

- Do you bill for laboratory tests done by commercial laboratories? How do you break down the fees?

—Autism Research Institute, www.autism.com
/pro_questions.asp

276. By working with your pediatrician to identify the various symptoms of autism or related conditions, your child's teacher, family friends, and peers can work together to help adjust behavioral and social or communication skills that the child may be deficient in.

—www.adviceaboutautism.com/treating-autism-at-home.html

277. You will want to include your child's pediatrician in the overall treatment strategy (biomedical, educational, therapies, etc.). It is imperative that the pediatrician allows time for you to discuss concerns, and for them to devote the time to work with you in addressing those concerns.

278. When you consult an expert, notice whether the waiting room is friendly to an autistic child. It should not be too busy or noisy. There should be toys in the room that might interest an autistic child.

—Areva Martin, Esq., *The Everyday Advocate*

279. When discussing your son with your selected medical professionals, you need to be credible and informed in order to have people listen to you and respect what you say. Never let professionals intimidate you.

CHAPTER 26

Diet

280. Changing your child's diet is one or perhaps the most significant thing you can do to impact your child's health. The Gluten-Free/Casein-Free (GF/CF) diet is the most popular; we suggest removal of soy as well as soy has similar properties to casein. Beyond this, the Specific Carbohydrate (SCD) Diet has been effective for those children who did not respond sufficiently to the GF/CF.

281. Where diet is concerned, I suggest being careful that you don't remove all the child's motivators for the sake of the gut, and leave yourself with no way to connect or entice for the sake of the brain.

—Lynette Louise, MS, Board certified in
Neurofeedback by BCIA, NTCB

282. Put your son on an organic diet, and remove additives, preservatives, colorings, processed carbs, and sugars (and don't forget juice, which is usually mostly water and high fructose corn syrup). Instead, utilize complex carbs (slower absorption) and healthful proteins, then observe. This will provide clues on which diet to follow, and how strict implementation will need to be. This will also provide good clues for your nutritionist and medical team as to what strategies may work.

283. If you begin to suspect a particular food item might be impacting behavior, test. Give your son two weeks away from the item and observe the results. It will be another clue for your medical team. Don't forget to remind folks at school about this, and other food restrictions.

284. Fussy eating is a common problem. In some cases the child might be fixated on a detail that identifies a certain food. Hilde De Clercq found that one child only ate Chiquita bananas because he fixated on the labels. Other fruit such as apples and oranges were readily accepted when Chiquita labels were put on them. Try putting different but similar foods in the cereal box or another package of a favorite food. Another mother had success by putting a homemade hamburger with a wheat-free bun in a McDonald's package.

—Temple Grandin, PhD, author of *Thinking in Pictures* and *The Way I See It*; www.autism.com/ind_teaching_tips.asp

285. Want to save a bundle? Plant a garden! Even a small patio can grow plenty of money-saving and healthy food, plus it's great for the kids to learn! If you have room for a tree, make it something that fruits and feeds your family. Also, buy food in season because it's cheaper when it's abundant.

—TACA; gfcf-diet.talkaboutcuringautism.org /gfcfsf-diet-on-food-stamps.htm

286. You wouldn't let your typical child live on a diet of Goldfish crackers and Skittles. Your child with autism is no different.

—Judith Chinitz, MS, MS, CNC, author of *We Band of Mothers*

Note: Tips 287–300, 302–305, 307–313, 315, 319–321 and the lists on pages 140 and 143 are adapted from the chapter "Dietary Interventions for Autism," in *Cutting-Edge Therapies for Autism*, which is adapted from the *Encyclopedia of Dietary Interventions for the Treatment of Autism and Related Disorders* (2008) by Karyn Seroussi & Lisa S. Lewis, PhD (available at www. sarpsborgpress.com).

---

287. Children with autism as a group have notoriously poor nutrition coupled with vitamin and mineral deficiencies. This may be due, in part, to extreme eating habits (they are notoriously picky). Deficiencies are also likely due to the abovementioned tendency toward malabsorption. This is why physicians who specialize in the biomedical treatment of autism start out by addressing malabsorption issues, adding digestive enzymes to the diet, eliminating problematic foods (usually including gluten and casein), stabilizing the condition of the gastrointestinal tract by removing allergens and harmful organisms, and introducing nutrients not being properly absorbed and utilized by the body. This approach has resulted in significant improvement in cognitive function, and in some cases, a full recovery from many of the symptoms of autism, if not the underlying disorder.

288. This approach can be challenging for parents. Changes in diet and supplementation are not usually expensive, but can be hard to implement. There are no guarantees, but thousands of parents will tell you that it is worth the effort. Changes in behavior, improvements in bowel function, increased language, and decreased self-stimulation are common responses to biomedical interventions. But if you're going to do it, commit to doing it fully—halfway measures are unlikely to bring about improvement.

289. Most newcomers fear that dietary intervention will be an uphill battle. However, the ground does level off much sooner than you might expect. The diet will get much, much easier, and once improvement is evident, the support you receive from those around you—including spouses, doctors, and educators—will also increase.

290. Identify the Pre-Diet Diet: Make a list of all the foods your child likes and eats. What do they have in common? Perhaps they are all starchy, sweet, salty, dairy-based, or wheat-based. Perhaps they are all the same types of foods. A child eating ice cream, bananas, grapes, chocolate pudding, sweetened yogurt, apple juice, and ketchup is not eating a varied diet—he is eating milk and sugar. A child who only eats bagels, crackers, cereal, pretzels, and waffles is not eating a varied diet; he is mostly eating one food: wheat. Foods that are craved are highly suspect, especially dairy- and wheat-based foods. Next, make a list of your child's physical symptoms. Does he get rashes? Does he get red cheeks or red ears after meals? Is his stomach bloated? Does he have diarrhea or constipation? Is he insensitive to pain? Note how these symptoms are associated with food; for example, does your child get red cheeks shortly after eating a particular food? Are bowel problems associated with any particular types of food? Are his behaviors worse at certain times of day, before or after meals?

291. Begin giving a multivitamin and mineral formula that is both low allergen and free of gluten and casein (common additives in vitamins). There are several available that are appropriate for children with autism made by specializing companies.

292. Ask your pediatrician to do a blood test for celiac disease (CD) *before* removing gluten. To be thorough, they should check total IgA, gliadin IgA, and IgG, and tissue transglutaminase IgA. It is likely to come back negative, since the blood test for CD is targeting only one specific type of gluten allergy.

293. Commit to a three-month trial of dietary intervention. Join an online support group such as the one at www.GFCFdiet.com. Choose a date, planning a day or two's meals at a time.

294. Start a food diary—this will turn out to be an important tool and should not be overlooked. Get a spiral pad or notebook and list each food your child eats on the left side of the page. On the right side of the page, list any changes you observe. Make a note of things like aggression, crying, whining, red ears, itchiness, bowel changes, or sleep problems.

\

295. Remove all dairy products from the diet, and within a week or two, all gluten. Using sugars, rice, potatoes, and other starchy foods to achieve this transition may be necessary, but keep in mind that they will probably need to be reduced or even removed later on.

296. Consider removing soy and corn at the same time gluten is removed. Many parents have given up on the gluten-free diet because they saw no change or a regression in their children, after having substituted soy for milk or corn for gluten. These two foods are almost universally problematic when starting the diet. They can always be added back later on a trial basis.

297. It is common to see crankiness, regression, or withdrawal symptoms during these first few days. Stay the course, and let your child know that you mean business.

298. Keep it simple: Instead of providing homemade or commercially available chicken nuggets, teach your children to eat plain chicken that has been baked or broiled. Cut the chicken into child-friendly strips and serve with a simple dipping sauce that you can make from scratch, quickly and cheaply. Teach your children to eat fruits and vegetables that are raw or gently steamed, again, using a simple sauce at first if they won't even try them plain, or blending them into pasta sauce or soup.

299. For those who are willing to learn to follow some simple recipes at home, dietary intervention shouldn't increase your family's food bill by very much. In fact, it may save you quite a bit of money, since you are far more likely to pack healthy, safe foods before leaving the house, and far less likely to grab a meal at a fast-food restaurant.

300. Get support: Compile a few articles on diet that you can give family members, teachers, and other caregivers. Tell them what you are doing, and why. Ask for their support.

301. The Autism Research Institute has a sheet on their website that you can print and hand out to unsupportive teachers, neighbors, friends, and family members who might be tempted to sabotage the diet: www.autism.com/pdf/providers/GFCF_science.pdf.

302. Remember: Just because the child does not test positive for wheat and dairy allergy does not mean that these foods are tolerated.

303. Sometimes changing the diet can lead to striking results within a short period of time. Younger children who are drinking large quantities of milk or eating primarily dairy- or wheat-based foods might exhibit changes within a week. But for most, the change won't be apparent until a few weeks later—often after accidental ingestion, when there is a noticeable regression. You might notice changes within a few days, but if not, be patient.

304. For some children, it might be necessary to simultaneously remove other foods, especially soy, corn, and even rice. Some children will require the elimination of all complex carbohydrates and others will need to reduce oxalates.

305. Most cheese substitutes contain some form of casein. It can even be found in tuna fish and other canned foods. Many wheat-free cereals contain malt (from barley) and thus are not gluten-free. Chewing gum, stickers, Play-Doh—all of these can be sources of gluten and casein. In short, you need to be a detective and investigate everything that goes into your child's mouth. Remember that, especially with small children, nonfood items often end up there too. Just a trace can make a world of difference in your results.

306. Additionally, you might have heard recently of a study where researchers tested dozens of products labeled gluten-free, and found that 70 percent of them failed the test. What to do? Move away from all processed foods. Use "gluten/casein-free" processed products only as a stepping stone to a cleaner diet. There are also many alternatives to processed items; for instance, potato chips over all others. Just get the chips that only have potatoes as an ingredient along with a helpful oil such as avocado, oil, or canola. Salt should only be sea salt.

307. Experience has shown that most people on the autism spectrum will benefit from a diet that is strictly free of gluten and dairy; therefore, the removal of these should be considered the foundation for dietary interventions. Additional changes are almost always needed for optimum improvement, but one size does not fit all. Every parent's goal is to find the ideal removal or rotation of foods for their child that will provide maximum benefit without being unnecessarily restrictive.

308. The most commonly restricted foods include gluten, dairy, corn, soy, yeast, oxalates, sugars, and starches. Other principles might apply, such as the use of probiotic foods, healthy fats, organic foods, and the restriction of food additives and artificial colors.

309. Most people get the hang of the diet in a week or two, and many good substitutes are now available for traditional wheat products. There are commercially available gluten-free breads at many supermarkets and at all health-food stores. Crackers without wheat or gluten are also widely available, made from grains, rice, and even nuts. If your child likes pasta, there are many excellent gluten-free alternatives; they come in different shapes and sizes and can be used in any recipe. Gluten-free baking, once you get the hang of it, is an economical way to prepare your family's favorite baked goods at home.

310. Many children start the diet eating only breaded, fried "nuggets." You can prepare these by making your own breading out of acceptable cereals, flours, or ground nuts. Most commercially prepared and fast-food versions are unacceptable.

311. It is a good idea to learn to read labels, and to call companies for information whenever you are unsure about an ingredient or food.

312. Look for fruits that have no sulfites (added to preserve color and retard spoilage), especially if phenols are a problem. Be aware that raisins sold in canisters may have traveled down a conveyor belt that was dusted with flour to prevent the fruit from sticking together. Because the flour is not an "ingredient," it does not have to be listed on the package.

313. "Hidden" gluten can also be found in some unexpected places, such as the glue on envelopes, Dixie cups, ground spices (some use flour to prevent clumping), appliances, fast-food fryers, and tropical fish food.

314. If you're thinking, "But the only things my picky eater is willing to eat are gluten- and casein-based," you're not alone. In fact, these children are the likeliest responders. Some parents say, "I can't possibly consult a nutritionist or dietitian—my child is a picky eater." Professionals are trained to address picky eating— they don't often hear from parents of children who happily eat a wide array of healthy lean meats, fruits, and vegetables.

A List of Foods and Ingredients that Always Contain Gluten

- Barley
- Barley grass (can contain seeds)
- Barley malt
- Beer
- Bleached flour
- Bran
- Bran extract
- Bread flour
- Brewer's yeast
- Brown flour
- Bulgur (bulgur wheat/nuts)
- Cereal binding
- Chilton
- Club wheat
- Common wheat
- Couscous
- Dextrimaltose
- Durum wheat
- Edible starch
- Einkorn
- Emmer
- Farina
- Farina graham
- Filler
- Flour
- Fu
- Germ
- Graham flour
- Granary flour
- Groats
- Hydrolyzed wheat gluten
- Hydrolyzed wheat protein
- Hydrolyzed wheat starch
- Kamut
- Malt
- Malt extract
- Malt flavoring
- Malt syrup
- Malt vinegar
- Matzo semolina
- Mir
- Pasta
- Pearl barley
- Rice malt (if barley or Koji are used)
- Rye
- Seitan
- Semolina
- Semolina triticum
- Shot wheat (*Triticum aestivum*)
- Small spelt
- Spelt (*Triticum spelta*)
- Spirits (Specific Types)
- Sprouted wheat or barley hydrolyzed wheat protein
- Strong flour
- Suet in packets
- Tabbouleh
- Teriyaki sauce
- Textured vegetable Protein—TVP
- Triticale
- Udon
- Unbleached flour
- Vegetable starch
- Wheat flour lipids
- Wheat germ
- Wheat grass (can contain seeds)
- Wheat nuts
- Wheat protein
- Whole-meal flour

315. Getting Enough Calcium with the GF/CF Diet:

- Green vegetables such as kale, collards, and bok choy are excellent sources of calcium, with the added benefit of being low in oxalates (spinach, though high in calcium, should be avoided if oxalates are a problem).

- Certain fish, like salmon and perch, are also good sources of calcium, but take care to buy fish that is not high in mercury or other environmental toxins (the smaller ones).

- A mere tablespoon of molasses contains 172 mg of calcium (as well as iron), so if yeast is not a big problem, it is a good choice for sweetening baked goods.

- Some nuts, beans, and seeds (like sesame seeds) are rich in calcium, but they should be ground for best absorption.

- Finally, if a child will not eat enough nondairy sources of calcium, there are many good supplements available. Because vitamin D is required to properly absorb calcium, a good supplement will contain both.

316. To eliminate the chance of ingesting toxins via food, avoid toxic fish, especially those who are the larger, longer-living species such as swordfish, which wind up absorbing more of the mercury in the ocean. Others in the group include tilefish and marlin and shark. Check out the following site from the Natural Resources Defense Council for a more detailed list of fish with the most, and least mercury: www.nrdc.org/health/effects/mercury/guide.asp.

317. Consider seeing a nutritionist or dietitian trained in the implementation of diets that have been successful for some people with ASD. The Autism Research Institute (ARI) maintains a list on their website (www.autism.com) of professionals who have attended their nutrition seminars.

318. Remember the prime source of vitamin D (which stimulates the production and use of calcium in the body) is the sun. Get enough sunlight on your child each day, about fifteen minutes will do, and skip the sunblock during this time. Worried about the rays? Take your fifteen minutes in the early morning or late day when the sun is "weaker."

319. There are several packaged foods that surprisingly contain some form of milk protein, such as canned fish and bread. Even soy and rice cheeses generally contain some form of casein or sodium caseinate. It is imperative that you learn to read and understand labels, and that you continue to check them each time you buy a food.

Foods to Avoid

Foods to Avoid (Always Contain Dairy)	Foods to Be Wary Of (Often Contain Dairy)
• Butter	• Baked goods (even if GF)
• Cheese (all types)	• Bologna
• Skim milk	• Broth (canned)
• Whole milk	• Candy
• Buttermilk	• Canned foods
• Powered milk	• Salad dressings
• Evaporated milk	• Candies
• Condensed milk	• Cakes/cake mix
• Goat's milk	• Chewing gum
• Sheep's milk	• Chicken broth
• Casein/caseinates	• Creamed vegetables
• Lactose	• Margarine/buttery spreads
• Milk chocolate	• Mashed potatoes
• Yogurt	• Nougat/caramel/toffee
• Kefir	• Pudding/custard mixes
• Ice cream/ice milk	• Scrambled eggs
• Cream	• Soy cheese
• Sour cream	• Tuna fish (canned)
• Cottage cheese	
• Whey	

320. Keep in mind that "nondairy" does not mean milk-free. It is a term the dairy industry invented to indicate less than 0.5 percent milk by weight, which could mean fully as much casein as whole milk.

321. Some of the most popular autism-diet groups include:

- Gluten-Free/Casein-Free Diet (GF/CF): www. yahoogroups.com/group/gfcfkids
- The Specific Carbohydrate Diet (SCD): www.yahoogroups. com/group/pecanbread
- The Low Oxalate Diet (LOD): www.yahoogroups.com/ group/Trying_Low_Oxalates
- The Feingold Diet: www.yahoogroups.com/group/ Feingold-Program4us
- The Body Ecology Diet: www.bedrokcommunity.org

322. A treatment based on negative reinforcement is used with children whose inappropriate behavior is maintained by escape from presentations of liquids or solids. Typical negative reinforcement-based treatments include providing a break following appropriate behavior (e.g., acceptance, swallowing) and elimination of escape for inappropriate behavior. A treatment based on positive reinforcement is used with children whose inappropriate behavior is maintained by attention. Typical positive reinforcement—based treatments include providing attention or tangible items following appropriate behavior (e.g., acceptance, swallowing) and the elimination of attention for inappropriate behavior.

—Dr. Petula Vaz and Dr. Cathleen Piazza, *Food Selectivity and other Feeding Disorders in Autism, Cutting-Edge Therapies for Autism,*

323. The Six Essential Healing Program Diets
- The Gluten-Free, Casein-Free Diet, or GF/CF Diet (best to remove soy as well)
- The Specific Food Reaction Diet
- The Anti-Yeast Diet
- The Anti-Hypoglycemia Diet
- The Specific Carbohydrate Diet
- The Low-Oxalate Diet

—Kenneth Bock, MD, *Healing the New Childhood Epidemics*

324. To achieve a therapeutic effect from nutrition, relatively high levels of specific nutrients are needed. These high levels are generally not attainable just from the daily diet. For example, to achieve a relatively high dosage of vitamin C, such as 500 mg [the amount found in many vitamin C tables or capsules] a person would need to eat ten oranges.

—Kenneth Bock, MD, *Healing the New Childhood Epidemics*

325. It might be hard to locate a substitute for the milk your child loves, although many children do adapt to the gluten-free, casein-free (GF/CF) soy, potato, almond, and rice milk substitutes available. Many parents provide vitamin and calcium supplements to their children on the diet.

—www.autismweb.com/diet.htm

326. Foods that *can* be eaten on a gluten-free, casein-free (only) diet include rice, quinoa, amaranth, potato, buckwheat flour, fruits, oil, vegetables, beans, tapioca, meat, poultry, fish, shellfish, teff, nuts, eggs, and sorghum, among others.

—www.autismweb.com/diet.htm

327. Use only sea salt, and as little as possible. Common refined table salt contains aluminum. Yes, aluminum. It is used to cut the salt and keep it from sticking. Needless to say, this is quite unhealthy, and it's good to know that aluminum enhances the toxicity of other toxins.

328. While it might be unrealistic to expect your entire family to take this novel dietary path, the benefits of introducing everyone to more whole foods should be obvious. We began the GF/CF (gluten-free, casein-free) diet as a family so that [our daughter] wouldn't feel singled out or deprived.

—Julie A. Buckley, MD, *Healing Our Autistic Children*

329. There is no one diet that works for everyone, and you need to consider all dietary intervention carefully, based on your child. Use the interventions discussed here as the foundation, and build wisely upon it. Don't diet-hop and -shop—work with a knowledgeable practitioner in developing the best diet for your child, one that might incorporate elements from a number of known diets. Stick with the plan—with most advanced dietary interventions, it takes months (typically a minimum of three) to see significant improvement. Don't throw in the towel—dietary changes are one of the most difficult things we do; most of our children are already on self-restricted diets, and much revolves around food preparation and consumption, so it's easy to be discouraged. Ask for help when you need it! Don't make decisions about diet rashly or in isolation—coordinate all diet plans with your medical-care plans to maximize outcomes of all interventions.

—Kelly Barnhill, CN, CCN, Director of the Nutrition Clinic at Thoughtful House Center for Children

330. Don't dismiss trying a special diet because it's "too much work." It's a lot easier to bake some damn muffins than to have a child with autism.

—Judith Chinitz, MS, MS, CNC, author of *We Band of Mothers*

CHAPTER 27

Biomedical Treatments

Biomedical treatment for autism refers to the Autism Research Institute's (ARI) Defeat Autism Now! (DAN!) project. The approach involves trying to treat the underlying causes of the symptoms of autism, based on medical testing, scientific research, and clinical experience, with an emphasis on nutritional interventions. Many of the treatments have been found by listening to parents and physicians.

—Jane Johnson, Managing Director, Autism Research Institute

We look at the body from the biochemical perspective and attempt to treat the root cause rather than just patch a Band-Aid on the symptoms. Psychotropic medications (Prozac, etc.) will not heal your children; they will only mask the symptoms of their poor health. Biomedical intervention is not alternative. We run tests to determine the source of dysfunction, and then we treat.

—Bryan Jepson, MD, Medical Director, Thoughtful House Center for Children

331. To find more information and a list of ARI/DAN! Practitioners in the U.S., visit www.Autism.com

—Jenn Gross, OTR/L

332. Make sure your child's doctor is one whom you are comfortable with, and who specializes in treating the medical needs of kids with autism. He or she should be regularly attending autism medical conferences to keep up-to-date, and ideally be someone who regularly communicates with other autism experts. Parents must educate themselves and exercise caution when selecting a clinician.

333. When beginning the biomedical approach, take it in a stepwise manner so that you can keep proper track of therapies and their impact. Additionally, you do not want to inundate yourself or your child.

334. Although many tips in this book state that early intervention brings better outcomes, this should not, and is not meant to, discourage those of you whose children are older (which includes myself). Biomedical and every other therapeutic approach can be started at any age, including teens and adults. We have heard many stories of people with autism at all ages showing significant improvement with various therapies.

335. Find a biomedical "maven," someone already ahead of you on the learning curve. This could be another parent you know, someone from a parent social group, or your son's school. If you cannot find someone nearby that you trust, you can contact organizations such as the National Autism Association (NAA), Talk About Curing Autism (TACA), or Generation Rescue (GR). All have lists of parents who are biomedical mavens and donate their time to talk to parents who are new to the approach. Check out the NAA and GR sites. NAA calls their mavens Naavigators and GR calls them Rescue Angels.

336. Of course, you can educate yourself, which you need to do anyway. For some places to start, check out the recommended reading list starting on page 453.

337. There is an overall series of steps which the DAN! practitioners tend to follow. For your information, we have adapted Dr. Robert Sears's list from *The Autism Book*:

- Step 1—Testing
- Step 2—Diet changes to clean up his gut/diarrhea/ constipation
- Step 3—Nutritional supplementation
- Step 4—Treating yeast, intestinal infections as indicated from the testing step
- Step 5—Begin methylation via B12 shots or nasal spray
- Step 6—Treat any viral infections indicated from testing
- Step 7—Treat other associated medical problems (i.e., immune dysregulation or chronic GI yeast infections)
- Step 8—Detoxification therapy
- Step 9—Hyperbaric oxygen therapy

338. When beginning the GF/CF diet, remove casein first, as it is easier to eliminate from your diet than gluten. There are many good milk substitutes, and casein is not in as many foods; it's easier to ferret out. Again, you will have to become a good label detective to eliminate all sources of casein. When beginning to remove milk/dairy products from your diet, remember to supplement with calcium!

339. Soy? While soy in some cases may be a good substitute for milk, it does have some casein-like properties, which make it a candidate for removal after gluten. Best to avoid from the get-go.

340. When beginning to remove casein and then gluten (and perhaps other foods), phase out the products. First, it will make things easier to take for you and your child, and second, it gives you time to learn the various sources of these products in your diet. You'll be surprised and perhaps shocked at the extent of their use in the Western diet.

341. Depending on your child's sensitivity, you may need to get extreme in removing the products; if so, don't forget products like soaps, shampoos, and such.

342. Don't force picky eaters to eat. Just prepare the healthy foods and serve. Give it a day or two while keeping them hydrated. Most kids will begin to try what is in front of them as soon as they grow hungry. For those who do not, a strategic retreat may be in order, but give it those couple of days first. If it's no go, fall back, look for more alternatives, and try again a week later. If after a few attempts you are having no luck, consult a nutritionist, and, of course, other parents!

343. Most pros think you should give the diet a good six months. Personally, I am always learning about new alternatives, and I feel that six months may be a bit short, given that it will likely take you weeks just to clean up the diet. It's best to adopt the diet as a family and look to make constant improvements to it over time; you'll all feel and perform better in the long run!

344. To this end work to eliminate not only gluten and casein but also any artificial ingredients and sugars. Focus on eating organic and local.

345. Keep a diary, including what your child takes and ultimately eats, along with results such as hyperactivity level, bowel movements, stimming, and any tantrums.

346. From my experience, the behavioral and cognitive symptoms of many ASD children can be noticeably improved with proper bio-medical treatments. Sometimes the improvement is dramatic enough for a child to lose his or her ASD diagnosis.

—Jaquelyn McCandless, *Children with Starving Brains*

347. Before starting down this road, remember that most recoveries and improvements have taken considerable time. In many cases your child has been "sick" for a while, and there is no quick fix. Think of biomedical therapy as a marathon that will take considerable time and perseverance, so you need to pace yourself. And, most important, a marathon is much more mental than physical; mental strength is the key. There is no magic bullet.

348. Look for the trend. During the course of biomedical treatments, you will see some progression and possibly some regression. Autism is a chronic condition, so it's often two steps forward, and one back. Focus on the trend: Are you better this year compared to last year? Day to day is too variable; think month to month and year to year. Compare your son to how he was this same time last year, as weather, allergens, and temperatures can cause interim disruptions; year to year is the best indicator of a favorable trend.

349. Don't count on yourself to notice and remember progress—or lack thereof—keep careful notes. You'll often find yourself thinking, "Wow—I had forgotten that he used to do that."

350. Younger kids may respond quicker, but do not give up if they don't. Also, kids are never too old to start. Plus, you never know what treatments will become available; there are new therapies to try every year. Keep breathing and moving forward!

351. Attend a medical conference, such as one of the two conferences held annually on each coast by the Autism Research Institute (once known as the Defeat Autism Now! conferences). ARI also posts their conference presentations online for free at www.autism.com. There is also AutismOne in Chicago each May, as well as many helpful regional conferences. These conferences usually have parent training seminars and explore the latest biomedical research and treatments. It's also great to hear success stories, learn from others, make new contacts, and renew old friendships. Some conferences are autism-friendly for the kids.

352. Much of what is required of you will be a significant effort to help with treatment—without understanding a treatment; you might give up too quickly.

353. Do your own research, and do not rely solely on your doctor to know all. You as a parent are the key advocate for your son, and you need to be active in the treatment process. Learn all there is to know about autism, and share it with the doctor(s). This education will help you understand the complex treatment process and keep you on task during difficult periods. You might have a great doctor, but no one cares as much as you do about the health of your child.

354. Be aggressive early. You have the best chance of helping your child when they are very young, so don't put off treatments. You don't ever want to look back and say, "If only . . ."
—Judith Chinitz, MS, MS, CNC, author of *We Band of Mothers*

355. When it comes to treatment for your child: If it can't hurt, and it could help, then do it. If it *can* hurt, then weigh the possible risks against the possible rewards. If the latter is heavier, then do it.
—Judith Chinitz, MS, MS, CNC, author of *We Band of Mothers*

356. The best laboratory is your child (according to Dr. Sidney Baker). The only way to really know if a treatment is going to work is to try it. We don't have the lab testing to predict individual reactions.
—Judith Chinitz, MS, MS, CNC, author of *We Band of Mothers*

357. Become an educated consumer; familiarize yourself with PubMed, the government's database of published research (www. ncbi.nlm.nih.gov/sites/entrez?cmd=search&db=pubmed). When considering a possible treatment, search PubMed first and weigh the evidence.

358. When beginning biomedical therapies, it's best not to begin everything at once. Try to phase things in over the course of weeks and months so that you can determine what might and might not be working. If you start too much at once, you will not know what is working or what could be causing problems.

359. Children already affected by autism can and do recover or significantly improve when a combination of biomedical and behavioral/educational therapies are employed. Doreen Granpeesheh, PhD, BCBA-D, founder and executive director of the Center for Autism and Related Disorders, agrees: "While behavioral/educational and biomedical practitioners have individually helped provide successful treatment models for autism, working together, these interventions have led to the best possibilities for successful outcome."
—Teri Arranga, "Afterword," *Cutting-Edge Therapies for Autism*

360. Keep some sort of journal of therapies and treatments along with reactions. We have a spreadsheet for this that you can download at www.skyhorsepublishing.com/Therapy_Logbook.xls. Update this (or a similar log) daily, and over time, you will be able to see what is working, and share this information with your doctor and therapists.

361. Continue to keep good records of the improvements you see in your child's behaviors, as they are probably the most significant measure of any therapy's effectiveness.

—Julie A. Buckley, MD, *Healing our Autistic Children*

362. Two steps forward, one step back—most children with autism have progress followed by plateau or regression; it's best to look for the overall trend.

363. The four body systems most profoundly affected in autism are the metabolic, neurologic, immune, and gastrointestinal systems. These organ systems are probably the most poorly understood and the most complicated of any in our body, and they're also the most tightly integrated. For instance, more than 70 percent of the immune system is housed in the gastrointestinal tract, so you can't have a problem in one and not the other. All of the neurotransmitters (the chemicals in your brain) also exist in the gastrointestinal system, where they have separate roles. The GI system is one of the main barriers against neurotoxins. Everything is tightly connected.

—Bryan Jepson, MD, Medical Director,
Thoughtful House Center for Children

364. When giving supplements, it's best to teach your son to take pills/capsules, but in the interim, utilize liquids, powders, and chewables as available (most come in multiple formulations). Anything in a capsule can be mixed into food or drink.

365. What if your kid doesn't swallow pills? There are two important keys to success with this, the roux and the meat injector! Empty all your capsules into a small cup with highish sides (I use a 3 oz. Tupperware container), add any additional powders. Then add a tiny bit of liquid (I use filtered water or liquid molybdenum, depending on whether it is morning or evening)—just enough to make a roux (or thick paste), if you add too much liquid, the powders will clump and you will have a mess. Stir it thoroughly so it has an even consistency then add more water to almost fill the cup. Next comes the meat injector! Use a meat injector instead of a syringe (a syringe is at most 2T, a meat injector holds much more liquid)—you can purchase one at Bed Bath and Beyond or any store that carries cooking tools. Remove the needle, suck up the supplement stew and squirt it into your child's mouth.

—Peggy Lowery Becker, mom of an 11-year-old ASD boy

366. Watch the use of digestive enzymes, as they will break down probiotics; be sure to allow at least an hour between the two.

367. Likewise, zinc could interfere with the absorption of other minerals and some vitamins; give zinc a window of an hour or two.

368. To encourage your son to take pills/capsules: Use rewards to entice him to take his caps. Our kids usually have something they go absolutely bonkers over, so use it for good. You should also be firm about taking the caps; let him know that it will happen. It's not open to negotiation. To do this, don't try and fool him by hiding the cap in applesauce. I give Alex his supplements on top of the applesauce, so he knows what he's getting; the applesauce is just there to help make it easier.

369. If using powders or breaking open caps, you can mix into foods or try making a smoothie. It's a good way to get some nice antioxidant berries and other good stuff down with the supplements at the same time.

370. Some prescribed meds may only be available compounded, or they are easier to use in a compound form. Just remember that if you have Medicaid for your son, the compounding pharmacy has to be in your home state, or else Medicaid will not cover it (it's a state program).

371. Activated charcoal. AC lessens the die-off's associated with antifungal treatments and other antioxidant products. AC also serves to help with any GI disturbances, use it yourself and see! Just remember to give two hours before or after other meds/ supplements, as it will not discriminate in what is absorbs and removes.

372. Home Remedies: Epsom salt baths act as a natural detoxifier and also aid in constipation and help calming! The one occasional negative can be dry skin; if your child experiences dry skin, just add some baking soda to the mix.

373. Check out http://Autism-Conferences.com for a list of biomedical conferences around the nation. Attend one and learn; make contacts; get inspired!

374. When dealing with constipation, remember one good "cleaning" is *not* all it takes. In most cases it took your child years to develop the condition, you need to get him regular for months to shrink the colon back to size!

375. For handling constipation there are a number of reliable and safe non-medical alternatives including supplementing magnesium (consult a physician for dosage), aloe juice (pour a little into the morning OJ) and Fruit-Eze, which is a prune, raisin, and date jam. If your child doesn't like the taste you can cover with something like peanut butter or syrup.

CHAPTER 28

The Metabolic System

376. Many of the metabolic abnormalities and susceptibilities that we commonly see in autism can be explained after examining the effects of acquired or inherited abnormalities in methylation and detoxification pathways. It's interesting to note that nutritional supplements associated with an improvement in autistic symptoms, either anecdotally or in the medical literature, happen to support normal function of these pathways. These include folinic acid, DMG, TMG, methylcobalamin, zinc, vitamin B6 (or P5P), digestive enzymes containing DPP-IV, GSH, cysteine (as N-acetyl cysteine), sulfate, and metallothionein-promoting amino acids.

—Reprinted by permission of the publisher. From Bryan Jepson, M.D., and Jane Johnson, *Changing the Course of Autism: A Scientific Approach for Parents and Physicians*, Boulder, CO: Sentient Publications. Copyright © 2007 by Bryan Jepson and Jane Johnson. All rights reserved.

377. Mitochondrial disorders often need specialized support, such as high doses of Coenzyme Q-10, although the actual deficiency that needs to be treated will depend upon what is actually wrong with the mitochondria. If these disorders are not treated early, then the person frequently will be very low-functioning in life and communication skills. Stroke in utero (like cerebral palsy) is one of those cases where HBOT can be beneficial.

378. Though [methyl-B$_{12}$] shots are initially feared by most parents, they soon learn that the shots are nearly painless, easy to administer, and give the greatest number of clinical responses when compared to oral, nasal, or transdermal routes of administration.

—Dr. James Neubrander, "Methyl-B$_{12}$: Myth or Masterpiece," *Cutting-Edge Therapies for Autism*

379. For children with autism, the results of transmethylation are increased language, focus and attention, awareness, cognition, independence, socialization and interactive play, appropriate emotional responses, affection, eye contact, and improvements in gross and fine motor skills.

—Dr. James Neubrander, "Methyl-B$_{12}$: Myth or Masterpiece," *Cutting-Edge Therapies for Autism*

380. I consistently find that the injectable form of methyl-B$_{12}$ is far superior to any other route of administration when one considers the percentage of children who respond, the intensity of each response, and how many responses each child exhibits.

—Dr. James Neubrander, "Methyl-B$_{12}$: Myth or Masterpiece," *Cutting-Edge Therapies for Autism*

The following is adapted from Dr. Richard E. Frye, "Mitochondrial Dysfunction," *Cutting-Edge Therapies for Autism*:

- Individuals with mitochondrial dysfunction should avoid physiological stressors.
- Patients should avoid fasting, extreme cold or heat, sleep deprivation, dehydration, and illness.
- If an individual with mitochondrial dysfunction becomes sick, there should be aggressive control of fever and hydration. During illness an individual with mitochondrial dysfunction should be closely monitored and provided intravenous hydration with carbohydrates if necessary.
- Certain drugs and environmental toxins which depress mitochondrial function should be avoided. Common toxins that inhibit mitochondrial function include heavy metals, insecticides, cigarette smoke, and monosodium glutamate. Common drugs that inhibit mitochondrial function include acetaminophen, nonsteroidal anti-inflammatory drugs, alcohol, some antipsychotic, antidepressant, anticonvulsant, antidiabetic, antihyperlipidemic, antibiotic, and anesthetic drugs.
- For some patients an overnight fast can be enough to destabilize mitochondrial function.
- Such patients can be treated with complex carbohydrates such as corn starch before bedtime. Some can be awakened in the middle of the night for a snack, while others might require a feeding tube to receive feeding overnight.
- Other patients respond to high-fat diets such as the ketogenic diet.

- Some patients respond to medium chain triglyceride oil supplementation, since these fats do not require carnitine to be transported into the mitochondria.
- Most vitamins are well tolerated, even at high doses. Some children with autism might have behavioral side effects from some vitamins. Thus, it is important to start vitamins one at a time, so that any side effects can be linked to a particular vitamin.
- Levocarnitine is linked to behavioral disturbances, especially in children with fatty acid abnormalities.
- Pyridoxine has been suggested to result in peripheral neuropathy at high doses.
- Children should be carefully monitored when the ketogenic diet is started, as the diet can worsen the metabolic acidosis associated with mitochondrial dysfunction.

CHAPTER 29

The Neurological System

381. While autism has been viewed as a brain disease for many decades, surprisingly little is actually understood about the brains of autistic patients. Various studies have looked at the structural and physiological differences in the autistic brain, but the results are inconsistent. This probably reflects the differences among subgroups of children with autism, all labeled with a common behavioral symptom complex but possibly stemming from different etiologies.

—Reprinted by permission of the publisher. From Bryan Jepson, M.D., and Jane Johnson, *Changing the Course of Autism: A Scientific Approach for Parents and Physicians*, Boulder, CO: Sentient Publications. Copyright © 2007 by Bryan Jepson and Jane Johnson. All rights reserved.

382. We think that the inflammatory process in the bowel may result in secondary inflammation in the brain. This is an important study that has come out recently: "Neuroglial Activation and Neuroinflammation in the Brain of Patients with Autism." Diana Vargas documented that autistic individuals have inflammation in the brain. This was one of the first studies to show this, because the inflammation doesn't show up on MRIs or CAT scans, but it does show up on biopsies of the brain (samples were taken from autistic individuals who had died.) The pattern of the inflammation is not consistent with the brain as the primary source. This is critical, because it suggests that the inflammation is starting somewhere else and the brain is a secondary target organ, not the primary source. If we can isolate the primary source, we have a target for treatment.

—Bryan Jepson, MD, Medical Director, Thoughtful House Center for Children

CHAPTER 30

The Immune System

383. There's a great body of evidence in the literature documenting immune dysregulation in autistic children leaving them prone to infection, chronic inflammation, and autoimmune reactions; it can affect any organ system, but the brain and the GI tract seem to be the worst hit. These immune system issues haven't been traced to a single underlying abnormality, and aren't always consistent among children on the autism spectrum. Just as there are subgroups based on behavioral characteristics, there appear to be subgroups within the autism spectrum related to the type and severity of immune abnormalities.

—Reprinted by permission of the publisher. From Bryan Jepson, M.D., and Jane Johnson, *Changing the Course of Autism: A Scientific Approach for Parents and Physicians,* Boulder, CO: Sentient Publications. Copyright © 2007 by Bryan Jepson and Jane Johnson. All rights reserved.

384. Autistic children have abnormal immune function, including low natural killer cell function and a TH1/TH2 imbalance. This means that affected children are much more likely to develop allergies and antibodies and a lot less able to kill off infections. They have chronic inflammation and autoimmune reactions. Many of them have eczema, chronic runny noses, ear infections—they seem to be sick all the time. I also see kids on the other end of the spectrum who never get sick. Even though the rest of the family is sick, they're fine. This suggests a hyper-immune state. These are the kids who are more likely to have autoantibodies. The body attacks itself because the immune system is on hyperdrive.

—Bryan Jepson, MD, Medical Director, Thoughtful House Center for Children

385. In an unstimulated state, individuals with autism have higher levels of proinflammatory cytokines (chemical messengers of the immune system) than control groups.

> —Dr. Mary Megson, "Viruses and Autism,"
> *Cutting-Edge Therapies for Autism*

386. With stimulation of the immune system (i.e., with the introduction of pathogens), individuals with autism spectrum disorders (ASDs) have markedly higher levels of proinflammatory cytokines than controls.

> —Dr. Mary Megson, "Viruses and Autism,"
> *Cutting-Edge Therapies for Autism*

387. Specific proinflammatory cytokines that have been found to be high in people on the spectrum include tumor necrosis factor-alpha (TNF-α) in both the blood and the gut; interferon-gamma (IFN-γ) in both the blood and the gut; and higher levels of interleukin-12 (IL-12) in the blood.

> —Judith Chinitz, "Helminthic Therapy,"
> *Cutting-Edge Therapies for Autism*

388. Individuals with ASD have lower levels of regulatory cytokines (those chemicals that turn off inflammation) like interleukin-10 (IL-10) than control groups.

> —Judith Chinitz, "Helminthic Therapy,"
> *Cutting-Edge Therapies for Autism*

389. Children might acquire viral infections at birth, in the perinatal period and beyond. Signs of viral infections in children with autism, due to increased Th2 response and immune suppression, are often not the usual signs of acute infection: nasal congestion, fever, cough, and/or nausea and vomiting. Chronic viral infections cause other symptoms: low endurance, rashes that come and go, and prolonged or intermittent low-grade fever. The children tire easily, have chronic congestion after allergy elimination, and are irritable.

—Dr. Mary Megson, "Viruses and Autism,"
Cutting-Edge Therapies for Autism

390. With autism, it is important to recognize that the effects of a particular virus might be far from the area of infection. For example, the antibody to measles cross-reacts with intermediate filaments.

—Dr. Mary Megson, "Viruses and Autism,"
Cutting-Edge Therapies for Autism

391. Another important defense against viral infections includes eating a healthy diet, getting adequate sleep and exercise, and avoiding stress in the child's life.

—Dr. Mary Megson, "Viruses and Autism,"
Cutting-Edge Therapies for Autism

CHAPTER 31

The Gastrointestinal System

392. Children with autism frequently have gastrointestinal problems, particularly constipation and diarrhea. When a child has GI symptoms, we generally find inflammation somewhere along the GI tract, but particularly in the terminal ileum, on endoscopy as well as biopsy. Many autistic children have evidence of abnormal intestinal permeability, or what we call "leaky gut." We continually find inflammatory bowel disease that is different from Crohn's disease and ulcerative colitis.

—Bryan Jepson, MD, Medical Director,
Thoughtful House Center for Children

393. Undiagnosed abdominal issues are the cause of many of the behavior symptoms of autism. If you imagine yourself as a nonverbal or poorly communicative individual who has chronic or intermittent abdominal pain, a lot of your behaviors are going to look pretty autistic. One example is abnormal posturing. We see some children go to great lengths to put pressure on their lower abdomen. They'll lie on the corner of a table or the arm of a sofa for hours. This was once considered an autistic behavior, but we now know that it's done exclusively to ease pain. What we've learned is that when you treat the abdominal symptoms, a lot of what were considered autistic behaviors disappear.

—Bryan Jepson, MD, Medical Director,
Thoughtful House Center for Children

394. If your child has frequent nighttime awakenings and/or wettings, they should have a full GI workup; nighttime awakenings can mean reflux, and wettings can mean allergies.

395. The presence of chronic (i.e., long-standing) GI symptoms demands medical evaluation. The fact that the child has autism is merely an interesting sidebar item. The symptoms typically consist of any (or all) of the following:

- abdominal pain
- diarrhea (defined as unformed stool that does not hold its own shape but rather conforms to the shape of the container/nappy/diaper that it is in)
- constipation (defined as infrequent passage of stool of any consistency or passage of overly hard stools regardless of frequency)
- soft-stool constipation
- painful passage of unformed stool
- rectal prolapse
- failure to maintain normal growth
- regurgitation
- rumination
- abdominal distention
- food avoidance

> —Dr. Arthur Krigsman, "Gastrointestinal Disease: Emerging Consensus," *Cutting-Edge Therapies for Autism*

396. Parents, physicians, and therapists must realize that difficult-to-treat ASD behaviors or behaviors that have not been responsive to standard behavioral interventions might be the sole manifestation of a GI diagnosis. This means that unprovoked aggression, violent behavior, and irritability might have an underlying GI cause, and this must be taken into consideration prior to the reflexive desire to begin a psychotropic drug such as risperidone (despite its FDA approval for the treatment of autism).

—Dr. Arthur Krigsman, "Gastrointestinal Disease: Emerging Consensus," *Cutting-Edge Therapies for Autism*

397. Gastroesophageal reflux disease, gastritis/gastric ulcer, and constipation are just three examples of GI diagnoses that are known to cause behavioral symptoms. In addition, poor focus and an inability to make significant academic or communicative progress despite intensive interventions might indicate the presence of treatable bowel disease that, once treated, can significantly improve the child's degree of disability.

—Dr. Arthur Krigsman, "Gastrointestinal Disease: Emerging Consensus," *Cutting-Edge Therapies for Autism*

398. Treatment of GI disease should follow established treatment protocols for the particular diagnosis.

—Dr. Arthur Krigsman, "Gastrointestinal Disease: Emerging Consensus," *Cutting-Edge Therapies for Autism*

399. GI diagnoses unique to ASD require further study to determine best treatment practices.

—Dr. Arthur Krigsman, "Gastrointestinal Disease: Emerging Consensus," *Cutting-Edge Therapies for Autism*

400. Like bacteria, some parasites are good and some are bad. And, like bacteria, some are perhaps meant to be in us. An absence of good bacteria in the gut will seriously compromise the health of the individual. More and more research suggests that an absence of good parasites is a major factor in the development of certain disorders.

—Judith Chinitz, "Helminthic Therapy," *Cutting-Edge Therapies for Autism*

401. Many children with autism have responded extraordinarily well to Trichuris suis ova (TSO, also known as helminthic therapy—or *worms*): improved digestive functioning, increased language and cognition, improved social skills, better mood and mood regulation, and more. The average amount of time it takes to begin to observe the changes is about twelve weeks. Some children, however, have certainly taken longer, even up to eighteen weeks. TSO is taken orally: Small vials of saline solution containing the invisible ova are drunk every two to three weeks. However, TSO is so expensive at the moment that it is beyond the reach of many families, especially considering that it must be done continuously.

—Judith Chinitz, "Helminthic Therapy,"
Cutting-Edge Therapies for Autism

402. Many doctors have noted that children with autism often have gut problems. Inflammation can be a major problem. Tissues that are inflamed are damaged. Damaged cells don't produce enzymes; therefore, many children with autism might present with deficiencies in some enzymes until the gut is healed and operating normally. Malabsorption might present as well. Food intolerance and outright food allergies might also manifest in these children.

—Dr. Devin Houston, "Enzymes for Digestive
Support in Autism," *Cutting-Edge Therapies for Autism*

403. Enzymes might be helpful in other ways for those with autism. Keeping the gut free of undigested material prevents putrefaction that might lead to pathogenic bacterial blooms and yeast problems.

—Dr. Devin Houston, "Enzymes for Digestive Support in Autism," *Cutting-Edge Therapies for Autism*

404. Gas and bloating might be minimized by using carbohydrase enzymes such as lactase and alpha-galactosidase. Some vegetables contain carbohydrates such as stachyose and raffinose that are difficult for humans to digest. The human gut lacks the enzymes to degrade carbohydrates that become a food source for gas-producing bacteria. Alpha-galactosidase enzyme supplements can make up for the deficiency and ease the bloating. Chronic diarrhea might also be helped through the addition of enzymes such as amylase and glucoamylase that degrade starchy foods.

—Dr. Devin Houston, "Enzymes for Digestive Support in Autism," *Cutting-Edge Therapies for Autism*

405. Give probiotics and prebiotics after a meal to maximize absorption, as stomach acid is then otherwise engaged.

CHAPTER 32

Seizures

The following tips are from Dr. Richard E. Frye, "Antiepileptic Medications," *Cutting-Edge Therapies for Autism*

406. **Seizure Syndromes:** Individuals with epilepsy related to a specific epilepsy syndrome, such as tuberous sclerosis, should be treated with AEDs that are effective for treating the specific underlying epilepsy syndrome.

407. **Emergency Seizure Treatment:** In many cases, rectal diazepam is very effective to treat prolonged seizure activity and may be prescribed to individuals with epilepsy or seizures that are at risk for such a prolonged seizure.

408. **Epileptic Encephalopathy:** AEDs have been more extensively studied for the classically recognized epileptic encephalopathies, specifically Landau-Kleffner syndrome and electrical status epilepticus during slow-wave sleep, than the less well-characterized syndromes such as subclinical electrical discharges. In general, the same medications appear to be just as effective for all the epileptic encephalopathies. Valproate has efficacy in some cases and may be the initial treatment choice. Occasionally, oxcarbazepine may be helpful for very focal electrical discharges. Immunomodulatory treatments, specifically steroids and intravenous immunoglobulin, may also be helpful adjunctive treatments for these syndromes. For electrical status epilepticus during slow-wave sleep, diazepam prior to sleep has also been used.

409. **Behavior and Mood Regulation:** Valproate and lamotrigine are particularly effective in mood regulation, while topiramate appears to be effective for reducing impulsivity and aggressive behavior.

410. **Migraine Headaches:** Valproate, gabapentin, and topiramate have been very effective in treating migraine headaches, with topiramate being particularly effective.

411. **Periodic Leg Movements during Sleep:** Gabapentin can be useful for treating period leg movements during sleep, especially if there is trouble with sleep initiation.

412. For the approximately one in five children with autism who suffer some sort of seizure disorder, it is important to note that marijuana is an excellent anticonvulsant, and was widely used as such in the last part of the nineteenth century and the early decades of the twentieth. Inhalation is not an option for children who suffer from autism; for these patients, the best route for administration is oral, in the form of cookies, brownies, tea, etc. Marijuana cookbooks are now available from which a variety of edibles that appeal to children can be found. With ingestion, the therapeutic effects will not appear before one and a half to two hours, but the advantage is that they last for many hours.

> —Dr. Lester Grinspoon, "Medicinal Marijuana: A Novel
> Approach to the Symptomatic Treatment of Autism,"
> *Cutting-Edge Therapies for Autism*

CHAPTER 33

To Medicate or Not to Medicate?

413. Medication can be used for the *short* term. Once your child starts a med, you aren't necessarily committing him to years of treatment. If you see positive results, your child can continue to take it for several months to a year, and then he can be weaned off it to see if it is still needed. Often a child matures or responds to all of his other therapies to the point that medication is no longer needed.

—Robert Sears, *The Autism Book*

414. Before accepting a drug prescription, ask a lot of questions, especially ones like: Are there any possible side effects? Will his sleep be affected? What is in the actual drug? How exactly does it work on my child's mind? Also ask about the success/non-success rate, as this is usually important when it comes to letting you know how effective the drug may be for your child's particular needs. Medications are not something to be treated lightly.

415. Signs that would alert you to the need for medication management include:

- Your child's safety is being questioned
- Increased episodes of physical aggression toward self and others
- Episodes of physical or verbal aggression are prolonged and not responsive to other intervention techniques
- Uncontrolled temper tantrums
- Fear that your child will hurt you or other members of your family or support team
- Increase in repetitive or stereotypic behaviors despite other interventions being in place
- Increase in anxiety, impulsivity, and inattention despite other interventions being in place

—Dr. Mark Freilich, "Pharmaceutical Medication
Management: The Why, When, and What,"
Cutting-Edge Therapies for Autism

416. Manifestations that may be helped by various pharmacologic agents include:

- Attention/distractibility/focus
- Repetitive/stereotypic behaviors
- Depression
- Anxiety
- Severe irritability
- Aggression/self-injurious behaviors
- Mood stabilization

—Dr. Mark Freilich, "Pharmaceutical Medication
Management: The Why, When, and What,"
Cutting-Edge Therapies for Autism

417. Antipsychotic drugs and mood stabilizers might help autistic patients who repeatedly injure themselves.

> —Dr. Lester Grinspoon, "Medicinal Marijuana: A Novel
> Approach to the Symptomatic Treatment of Autism,"
> *Cutting-Edge Therapies for Autism*

418. Anticonvulsants might be useful in suppressing explosive rage and calming severe anxiety.

> —Dr. Lester Grinspoon, "Medicinal Marijuana: A Novel
> Approach to the Symptomatic Treatment of Autism,"
> *Cutting-Edge Therapies for Autism*

419. The psychoactive medications that are most often used to treat autism are in the following major categories:

- Antidepressants
- Atypical antipsychotics (or neuroleptics)
- Anticonvulsants
- Stimulants (or ADHD medications)
- Anti-opioids
- Miscellaneous medications

> —Kenneth Bock, MD, *Healing the New Childhood Epidemics*

420. The Autism Research Institute has surveyed more than 27,000 parents since 1967; often-prescribed meds like Risperdal, Ritalin, and Prozac are by no means the most successful treatments. Before choosing psychotropic meds that often have unpleasant side effects, consider dietary intervention. Read ARI's survey: http://autism.com/pdf/providers/ParentRatings2009.pdf, and consider biomedical treatment. Make sure all educational therapies are appropriately implemented.

421. Symptoms such as aggression and self-injurious behavior are often responses to pain. Before assuming a psychological genesis, be 100 percent certain that your child is not in pain. In particular, stomach pain and/or gastroesophageal reflux should be ruled out.

422. Today there are many new drug treatments that can be really helpful to people with autism. These medications are especially useful for problems that occur after puberty. Unfortunately, many medical professionals do not know how to prescribe them properly.

—Temple Grandin, PhD, *Thinking in Pictures*

423. Before making the decision to medicate your son, work with your boy's team (professionals and family) to fully implement the suggested education plan and diet for a full six months.

424. Medication as a first line of action may allow the child to become more available to the positive effects of the various other treatment approaches that have been deemed appropriate. This can lead to a reduction in or the eventual elimination of medication.

　　—Dr. Mark Freilich, "Pharmaceutical Medication Management: The Why, When, and What," *Cutting-Edge Therapies for Autism*

425. If you choose to medicate, keep in mind that people with autism are often exquisitely sensitive to medication. Sometimes a surprisingly small dose can be effective. Be wary of professionals who don't understand this, and use a one-size-fits-all approach.

426. The process of determining the appropriate medication and the appropriate dosage cannot be completed overnight. The process will, at first, require weekly office visits (or at least weekly telephone communication) with the prescribing physician. If, at any point before finding the "optimal" dosage, the physician hands you a prescription and tells you that the plan is to administer the medication and return in a month's time, please consider another medication manager.

    —Dr. Mark Freilich, "Pharmaceutical Medication Management: The Why, When, and What," *Cutting-Edge Therapies for Autism*

CHAPTER 34

Preparing for that Inevitable Emergency Room Visit

427. Having a first aid kit at home is of absolute necessity, as is knowing how to use it! Take a class in first aid at your local fire house or medical facility and you may be able to save a visit to the doctor or other such facility that can be traumatic for our kids.

Bonus tip: To adjust to minor cuts and scrapes let your child play wear a band-aid now and then so the actually need is no big deal. Let them practice on you. Wear a band-aid yourself, or if there is a chronic issue try to mimic what they will have deal with so that they can become a bit more comfortable with the process.

428. When visiting the doctor or other related facility bring along something comforting for the child, such as a favorite toy or blanket or perhaps a video playing machine or small computer or book. Anything to keep busy and not have to focus exclusively on the stress of visiting a medical establishment. It may be useful to visit said establishment in advance to familiarize the child and remove one level of stress—the unknown.

Bonus tip: Watch some shows that have a nice comfortable perspective going to see medical personnel. Again this helps your child become familiar with the process and see that things will be OK.

429. Play doctor with your ASD child. Again, familiarizing him with what goes on in the medical office can help ease stress. Give him a play examination and let him give you one. Also when you visit the doctor or dentist, perhaps they can let your child listen to the stethoscope or hold a dental mirror and raise and lower the examination table/chair to gain their trust and interest.

Bonus tip: Walk around the facility with your kid. There will be restrictions to this of course, but in my experience staff at medical facilities were usually well-versed on autism and the anxiety the kids can experience. A little "tour" of the facility can help relieve at least some of the stress.

Chapter 35
DENTISTRY

430. When looking for a dentist for your ASD child search for those who specialize in ASD kids. If you do not have one of these specialists nearby focus on pediatric dentists as they will be more likely to have been exposed to special-needs kids and be better equipped to handle them. Some might even have specific days of the week when they only schedule children with special needs. Also don't neglect the all important parent network—ask the parents of your child's classmates for references.

431. Pretending to be examined yourself may help ease the anxiety your child feels upon dentist visits. If the dentist agrees, you may be able to interest your child in some of the equipment in the office; many kids may enjoy riding up and down on the examination chair and/or running the chair themselves.

432. If your child has an object that he particularly loves (a music player or clock, for example), bring one with you to the dental visit so that the dentist can incorporate that into the appointment.

—Ruby Gelman, DMD

433. I have found that short, more-frequent visits prove to be very successful in the dental office. I will recommend seeing autistic kids every two to four months, and at each visit, we do the same things we did at the visit before, while incorporating something new each time. Kids will remember things better from one visit to the next.

—Ruby Gelman, DMD

434. On June 12, 2008, the FDA admitted on its website that silver fillings in our teeth are toxic and harmful to our health, and that they "might have neuro-toxic effects on the nervous systems of developing children and fetuses." Avoid them. Likewise, research fluoride before allowing fluoride treatments or using fluoride toothpaste.

435. Be sure to choose a dentist who has experience treating kids who are on the autistic spectrum. The experienced dentist will be happy to speak to you prior to the appointment to formulate an appropriate treatment approach.

—Ruby Gelman, DMD

436. While many dentists recommend sedation for autistic kids, I do not believe it is appropriate if this is suggested without meeting your child in the dental office setting first.

—Ruby Gelman, DMD

CHAPTER 36

Treating the Common Cold and Flu

The tips in this chapter are adapted from the article "Treating the Common Cold and Flu: Special Considerations for ADHD, ADD, and ASD" by Kim Gould, RPh, MS, *The Autism File*, Issue 30, 2009.

Note: Evaluating treatment options is especially important in people with multiple sensitivities, such as those who have symptoms of autism spectrum disorders. Both the cold and flu are viral respiratory illnesses. The common cold may be bothersome, but the flu can lead to more dangerous and severe illnesses that can cause death in high-risk patients. Generally, we treat the symptoms of the cold or flu—not the virus itself.

437. Parents should check the active and inactive ingredients on product labels, as both may affect the well-being of a person with ASD.

438. Inactive ingredients such as preservatives, dyes, and other excipients can cause allergic reactions, such as rash, exacerbation of asthma symptoms, anaphylaxis, hyperactivity, and in some cases, upset stomach, and diarrhea. Some examples include:

- Preservative sodium benzoate, which can exacerbate asthma
- Preservative benzoic acid, which can cause hyperactivity
- Preservative parabens, which can lead to asthmatic reactions
- Sweetener aspartame, which can cause hives, swelling, and hyperactivity
- Sweetener sucrose, which can increase blood glucose and cause hyperactivity
- Sweetener saccharin, which can cause hives, itching, nausea, diarrhea, and other disturbances

439. When you have a prescription medication and would like to find out the inactive ingredients, there are a few ways. First, you can ask your pharmacist to look at the package insert. Under the title "description" at the very top of the insert, there is a list of all the ingredients in a manufactured product. Second, check a *Physicians' Desk Reference (PDR)*. The *PDR* is a compilation of package inserts printed as a book. Most libraries and large bookstores have a copy of the PDR. Unfortunately, only the most current high-volume prescription drugs are included in the book. Third, you can look online. Find the official website of the prescription drug you are checking on. Click on "health-care professional" and then go to the prescribing information section, which will bring up a copy of the package insert. The first item listed is the description, and the inactive ingredients are listed there.

440. When treating the symptoms of a cold or flu virus, it is best to look at each symptom and treat it accordingly. When you administer multisymptom-relief products, you may be giving unnecessary medications that may have unwanted side effects. So if you buy OTC medications to treat cold and flu symptoms, buy products that have single active ingredients and as few additives as possible.

441. Remember that colds and flu are viral infections. Therefore, antibiotics are not effective, and should not be taken to treat them. Antibiotics can cause resistant organisms, yeast overgrowth, and immune suppression.

442. When antibiotics are needed for secondary bacterial infections, probiotics should be used to help maintain a healthy gut. [Editor's Note: Probiotics should not be given at the same time as the antibiotic dose, but spaced midway between doses.]

443. The antibiotic Augmentin is commonly prescribed for children with ear infections. It has been reported that Augmentin should be avoided in patients with autism, Asperger's, ADD, or ADHD due to a potential adverse neurological effect caused by the clavulanate component of Augmentin.

444. The best approach in treating the symptoms is to look at each one individually and apply treatments according to each. At the first sign of symptoms (e.g., sore throat for cold), I like to start taking zinc and vitamin C, and I use an herbal blend drop containing echinacea, shiitake, and noni, which also boosts immunity.

445. Try some of the non-medicine interventions if you have not used them before. Nasal irrigation with saline solution (homemade or purchased) has become a popular alternative to decongestants. Warm liquids to drink, inhale, or bathe in are very comforting and therapeutic. A few drops of eucalyptus oil in a bath will help clear a stuffy nose and head.

446. Prevention is always the best medicine for colds and flu. Practice good hand washing and eating, drinking, and sleeping well; plus, a little knowledge about treatment options will go a long way.

447. Here are three ways to help alleviate congestion without using medications that may cause hyperactivity.

- Moist heat—Warm compresses to cheeks and sinuses (you can add one to two drops of tea tree oil or eucalyptus oil in the compress). Warm showers will also open airways and moisten thin sinus mucus.

- Drink more liquids—Drink at least six to eight cups of water each day to help liquefy the mucus that builds up. Warm water and herbal teas are more effective. Avoid liquids containing caffeine because these may cause dehydration.

- Nasal saline irrigation or saline nasal sprays—Scientific studies show saline nasal irrigation will thin mucus, decrease postnasal drip, and remove virus and bacteria particles from your nose. Xylitol nasal sprays can also be helpful in humidifying the nasal passage and decreasing nasal irrigation.

448. For a sore throat, use warm drinks and gargles. Drinking warm tea with honey (local honey may help with allergies; honey should only be given to children over the age of two) or gargling with warm honey/lemon/water or warm salt water.

449. Some alternatives to cough medicines include:
- Warm tea and honey.
- Slippery elm (available in lozenges with zinc). Slippery elm has received recognition from the FDA as a safe and effective treatment for cough and sore throat.
- Cough lozenges made from xylitol and honey (Ricola has a good-tasting drop).
- Peppermint thins mucus and will help loosen and break up the phlegm of a productive cough. It is soothing for dry coughs and sore throats. You can use either peppermint teas or candies (xylitol-based).
- Note: There are no OTC cough suppressants available for children under six years old, and those that are available should be used with caution for children under twelve years old.

450. When using antihistamines for runny nose, eyes, and sneezing, look for dye-free diphenhydramine (some products contain sodium benzoate and saccharin). You can also have it compounded with a prescription from your doctor. Newer non-drowsy antihistamines do not work for cold symptoms.

451. Quercetin is useful in stopping the production of histamine and inflammation; it is also a potent antioxidant. The University of Maryland has a great website for complementary medicine. A use and dosing guideline for Quercetin is available at www.umm .edu/altmed/articles/quercetin-000322.htm.

452.. When treating nausea, vomiting, and diarrhea, note the following:
- It is important to replace lost fluids and prevent dehydration. Include a variety of liquids (not cold, because that can upset the stomach more), such as water, broth, tea, and juices (watered down may be easier on the stomach).
- The BRAT diet is good until the system settles down (bananas, rice, pear sauce—instead of applesauce for the child who is limiting phenols—and gluten-free toast).
- Probiotics help to restore the normal flora of the gut. Again, just do not take at the same time as antibiotics.

453. To shorten the length of cold and flu symptoms, use vitamin C (ascorbic acid) and zinc (zinc lozenges).

CHAPTER 37

Anesthesia and Your Child

Your child might require anesthesia for dental or surgical procedures. Many people with autism have unusual responses to anesthesia. Ask to meet the anesthesiologist several days before the procedure. Print out and bring the advice of Dr. Louise Kirz, an anesthesiologist with two children on the spectrum (http://legacy.autism.com/families/life/kirz.htm).

The following tips are adapted from the article "Anesthesia and the Autistic Child" by Sym C. Rankin, RN, CRNA, MS, *The Autism File*, Issue 33, 2009.

454. Anesthesia is unavoidable for children who need to undergo surgical procedures. The goal in such cases is to minimize the risk. To do that, the anesthesia provider must be made aware of the unique problems your child has.

- Your child may have gastrointestinal dysfunction, immune system dysregulation, inflammation, mitochondrial dysfunction, heavy metal poisoning, oxidative stress, and chronic inflammation.

- Most importantly, your child probably has impaired detoxification systems and may not be able to metabolize drugs efficiently.

455. When your child is scheduled to undergo a procedure, consider discussing the following issues during the preoperative conference:

- Ask not to use nitrous oxide. Most of our kids have a documented B12 deficiency.

- Discuss specific medical and metabolic problems concerning your child. Tell your provider of any genetic, methylation, detoxification, and mitochondrial issues.

- Consider placement of an IV without sedation. Many of our children undergo multiple blood draws and intravenous treatments. If your child can tolerate an IV placement, let your anesthesiologist know that because the provider usually will not expect children to tolerate this procedure.

- Inform the anesthesia provider of all medications, supplements, and IgE allergies.

- Make sure the provider understands that your child has difficulty detoxifying drugs.

- Ask the provider to keep the anesthetic as simple as possible.

- Discuss any other drugs that might be given in conjunction with the anesthetics (e.g., acetaminophen, steroids, and antiemetics).

CHAPTER 38

Preventing Autism

Tips 456–484 are adapted from the article "Avoiding Autism" by Anju Usman, MD and Beth C. Hynes, JD, MBA, *The Autism File*, Issue 31, 2009.

456. Due to the symbiotic relationship between a mother and her developing fetus, care must be taken by the mom before, during, and after pregnancy (if nursing) to both avoid exposure to harmful elements and to promote optimal maternal detoxification processes so that the host body remains as clean an environment as possible, within which vigorous infant development can unfold. Considering this, basic principles to guide you in decision-making surrounding pregnancy are as follows:

- You are what you eat (and drink); therefore, make healthy choices in what you consume.
- Skin is the largest organ in the body, so be very careful about what you rub into yours and your baby's.
- Think beyond "green": What is "green" for the environment is not always what is healthiest for the body, but what is healthiest for the body is always "green."

Pre-Pregnancy

457. While planning a pregnancy, we recommend that you clean up any toxicity in your body and begin to follow a more organic, healthy lifestyle. Remember, the less toxic you are, the better it is for you and your future baby. Undertake a sequential detoxification program that targets the liver and colon; this type of program can take six months or more and should not be done while pregnant.

458. In a careful manner, with an experienced dentist, remove amalgams from your teeth, which also can take six months or more.

459. Take the time now to find organic, nontoxic makeup, hair, and body products that you like and start integrating them into your daily life.

460. Ask your doctor to run some tests to determine any additional specific supplementation you may need to optimize levels within your body.

461. Remove all harmful chemical cleaning agents from your cleaning routine at home and at the office, and instead use cleaning products labeled "Level 1" by the EPA. Do not forget to include products for dishwashing and clothing detergent in your cleanup, and avoid toxic dry cleaning as much as possible.

462. Improve your nutrition with a targeted vitamin supplementation program to include omega-3 essential fatty acids, sublingual methyl B-12, folinic acid, vitamin D3, zinc, and antioxidants.

463. Eat organic, hormone-free food and avoid consuming fish or foods with MSG or food dyes.

464. Drink organic green tea, filtered water, and antioxidant-rich organic juices while avoiding soda, carbonated beverages, and alcohol.

465. Use stevia, raw organic honey, and xylitol as sweeteners. Avoid any artificial sweeteners.

466. Go for walks and get some sunshine daily.

467. Cosmetics: Use aluminum-free natural deodorant, natural hennas to color hair, and avoid moisturizers or makeup with chemicals or parabens in them. Also avoid chemical dyes, perms, or other such hair treatments.

468. Use only chemical-free cleaning products in your home, and avoid using pesticides or chemicals to treat your lawn.

During Pregnancy

469. Avoid medications to the extent possible, as well as acetaminophen, because it hinders normal detoxification.

470. Add zinc, calcium, essential fatty acids, and prenatal vitamins to your daily supplement intake.

471. Discontinue use of nail polish and any makeup (including lipstick) products that contain parabens and other toxins.

472. Use fluoride-free toothpaste, as fluoride interferes with iodine metabolism.

473. Do yoga and engage in stress management techniques, such as massage and listening to soothing music. Do not, however, start a rigorous exercise program, sit in a sauna, or get dental work (not even cleanings).

474. Get the mercury-free RhoGAM if you need this intervention.

475. Eat fermented foods, cook with organic coconut oil, use organic raw apple cider as salad dressing, and consume healthy fats and cold pressed oil. Avoid fast food or seafood (especially tuna), and food packaged in plastic or Styrofoam. Do not use a microwave.

476. Use a corded headset while talking on a cell phone. Don't work with a laptop computer on your lap.

477. If you have amalgams and plan to nurse, you should send a sample of your breast milk to a specialty lab for heavy-metal testing.

478. If you plan to use formula, use those containing DHA (docosahexanenoic acid), an essential fatty acid critical to the healthy development of the central nervous system.

479. When introducing food, use organic baby food. Avoid the introduction of soy, gluten, or dairy until after the baby turns two years of age. After one year, supplement your baby's food with a quarter of a teaspoon of mercury-free cod liver oil.

480. For fevers over 101 degrees Fahrenheit, treat with a tepid bath or dye-free ibuprofen. Fevers, while nerve-wracking for new parents, are the response of a healthy immune system reacting to kill off an invading virus through heat.

481. Antibiotics should be used sparingly and only for confirmed bacterial infections (they do not alleviate viral infections). Remember, antibiotic use disrupts the normal gut flora and promotes the overgrowth of yeast and resistant organisms that, in turn, harms the optimal functioning of the immune system. Bear in mind that most ear infections are viral and are thus not treatable with antibiotics. Use homeopathic ear drops to help ease the symptoms associated with ear infections and colds.

482. Use an organic baby mattress, bedding, pillows, and hypoallergenic encasements. Avoid pajamas soaked in flame-retardant chemicals.

483. Bathe your baby daily in warm filtered water while avoiding soaps, moisturizers, or other "baby products" on the skin, as such items are unnecessary and contain harmful chemicals.

484. Feed your baby using glass bottles, avoiding plastic bottles and cups; also avoid microwaving formula or breast milk.

485. Vaccine Recommendations

- If your child has a fever, constipation, diarrhea, or other illness, hold off on the vaccination.
- If your child is on antibiotics, hold off on the vaccination.
- If your child has an immune system disorder, allergies, or if they had a reaction to an earlier vaccine, hold off on the vaccine and seek another opinion.
- Know what the possible reactions are to each vaccine given.
- Immediately report side effects to your doctor.
- Remember to ask for single-dose mercury-free vaccines.
- Break up the measles, mumps, rubella (MMR) shot and give those months apart.
- Check antibody titers before boosters, as they may not be necessary.

486. Here is the recommended vaccine schedule of Stephanie Cave, MD, DAN! practitioner, and vaccine expert:

- Birth: Hepatitis B (only if mom is Hepatitis B positive); otherwise, no vaccine shot
- 4 months: Hib, IPV
- 5 months: DTaP
- 6 months: Hib, IPV
- 7 months: DTaP
- 8 months: Hib
- 9 months: DTaP
- 15 months: Measles
- 17 months: Hib, IPV
- 18 months: DTaP
- 24 months: Prevnar (1 dose only)
- 27 months: Rubella
- 30 months: Mumps
- 4 years: Varicella (if not immune already)
- 4 to 5 years: Hepatitis B series
- 4 to 5 years: DTaP, IPV boosters
- 4 to 5 years: Test titers for MMR and do not give unless not immune. Immunize only for vaccines found to be negative.

487. If your pediatrician has a problem with these requests, choose another doctor.

SECTION 6

....

Supporting the Family Unit

There's turbulence ahead; please remember to secure your mask firmly before attempting to help others!

CHAPTER 39
Self-Care

488. Self-care is imperative for parents so that they are available to their child to help them develop the key components for social, emotional, and intellectual development, including the ability to focus and attend, engage, interact, and use ideas creatively and logically.

—Lauren Tobing-Puente, PhD, "Parent Support,"
Cutting-Edge Therapies for Autism

489. Accept that you are only responsible for the effort you expend in helping your child, not for the outcome, which is beyond your control.

—Carole Harris, Joshua's Mom

490. The 72-Hour Rule: Autism is hard, and we are human. We have a right to feel sorry for ourselves. When you need to, feel free to wallow in the deepest pool of self-pity you can muster. However, feeling sorry for ourselves accomplishes nothing. Therefore, only wallow for a maximum of three days. More than that, and it becomes habitual. Just seventy-two hours later, pick yourself up, get out there, and do something useful.

—Judith Chinitz, MS, MS, CNC, author of *We Band of Mothers*

491. It's essential that you take care of yourself and your needs, including giving yourself the time and space to grieve. You have lost the child you imagined you would have, and it's perfectly okay to mourn that loss. Mourn, but also discover the incredible new child you've been given. Eventually, those memories of that other child will fade and be replaced with the magnificent memories you will undoubtedly make.

492. Run! No not away from your troubles but as a way to deal with them. You need exercise to keep fit for battle, and nothing is easier, cheaper, or more fun than running. Running is also a bona fide stress reliever and provides an opportunity for your mind to organize its thoughts. Join a local running club or organization. Here in New York City we are blessed with the New York Road Runners, but there are many similar organizations around the country and if one is not near, start an affiliate!

Bonus Tip: When you get rolling with the running, drop the iPod and listen to yourself think!

Daily Double: Run with your son! What could be better? Get him involved, it can provide the same exercise, stress relief, and mental calming for him.

CHAPTER 40

Marriage Tips

493. A positive attitude will help. Today, marriages fall apart for a variety of reasons, and with an autistic child, however good and kind you might be in dealing with your child, it is exhausting, and the result is that it will take its toll on your marriage. So you need to adopt a positive frame of mind, and come up with solutions that will help both you and your spouse to spend quality time together.

—Abhishek Agarwal, www.health-whiz.com/555/index.htm

494. You will need to rediscover yourselves, and dwell on how you first met, what attracted you to each other, and try to remember each other's good points. Also, the autistic child needs to interact with other people as well, like a qualified nanny or a grandparent, even an uncle or aunt. This will definitely help the child to have a few other people in his life and be able to give you the break that you need, allowing you to spend more time with each other.

—Abhishek Agarwal, www.health-whiz.com/555/index.htm

495. Work together to save your marriage. Try to see what works best for your autistic child, and work together instead of blaming each other. Although it can be frustrating at times, you could agree to work on solutions that could help, and in the long run, it will be beneficial to both parents and child. Never try to medicate the child without first consulting a specialist. Prioritize your needs by keeping a certain time each week for time together as a family, especially if one parent spends most of their time with the child.

—Abhishek Agarwal, www.health-whiz.com/555/index.htm

496. You will also need to get as much help as you can to help you deal with each person's needs, and this is all the more necessary when you are looking after a child who is autistic. There might be a situation when neither of you feel that you are getting anything out of life because you do not have any time for yourselves, and so much of your time is spent caring for your child as a result of his special needs. In this case, it would be advisable to get the help of a counselor who can suggest solutions that will keep you both happy.

—Abhishek Agarwal, www.health-whiz.com/555/index.htm

497. Another important factor is the need to interact with other parents of autistic children; this way, you will be able to see how they deal with situations and exchange ideas which will help everyone. Always remember that you do not have to struggle alone; there is always help in the form of family, counselors, and fellow parents. By keeping the right perspective and a positive attitude, you can give your child the care and love he needs, as well as retain the spark in your marriage.

—Abhishek Agarwal, www.health-whiz.com/555/index.htm

498. Marriage is already stressful, and autism adds to the mix. Both parents will be stronger and better able to cope with life's tribulations if they stay together and work together. There are many battles ahead, so don't waste energy on infighting; it's destructive. Fight outward; be an army!

—Allison Edwards, Jon's Mom, UK Autism Campaigner for Cryshame (www.cryshame.org.uk) and Jabs (www.jabs.org.uk)

499. Don't turn to alcohol; it's not the answer to autism. Try a refreshing cuppa tea instead. It has fewer calories and it's far less explosive!

—Allison Edwards, Jon's Mom, UK Autism Campaigner for Cryshame (www.cryshame.org.uk) and Jabs (www.jabs.org.uk)

500. From a management perspective, it is most efficient to have one parent "in charge of"—to be the general, if you prefer—the autism battle. Many times one parent will be more focused on the effort and thus have more information at hand. That individual should make all the calls, while providing full disclosure to the other. The other parent should focus on other children in the family, or, in the case of a single child, a specific task—say, biomedical research, or planning family outings.

501. Forgive each other for not grieving the same way at the same time.

CHAPTER 41

Counseling and Support Groups

502. Individual counseling with a mental-health clinician allows opportunities for focusing on parents' own experiences and developing coping strategies that can help them manage their parenting stress and any symptoms of psychological distress. Here, they can specifically address their struggles in order to become more effective in their parenting roles and feel increased contentment overall.

—Lauren Tobing-Puente, PhD, "Parent Support,"
Cutting-Edge Therapies for Autism

503. Marriage counseling with a mental-health clinician who has a background in families of children with ASDs is often helpful for addressing issues within the marriage. Support for the siblings of children with ASDs is also important for addressing the impact on the entire family.

—Lauren Tobing-Puente, PhD, "Parent Support,"
Cutting-Edge Therapies for Autism

504. Parents should be as much the focus in treatment as the children themselves, as their well-being is critical to their ability to be a part of their children's therapy. The optimal functioning of the parents is essential if the treatment strategies are to be successfully implemented.

—Lauren Tobing-Puente, PhD, "Parent Support,"
Cutting-Edge Therapies for Autism

505. Parent support groups can be an amazing resource. Not only can they provide support as you raise your child with autism, but they can also provide a place to find out information regarding treatments other parents have tried, tips from other parents about traveling or community outings, after-school activities, and much more. Other parents know what you are going through; they are full of information about their own experiences, and are usually more than willing to share and help another parent out!

—Bonnie Waring, LMSW

506. Education regarding what is known about the cause(s) of ASDs is often crucial for parents who experience guilt and self-blame. Listening to others who have had similar experiences helps parents feel a sense of community, contrasting their experience of isolation from others.

—Lauren Tobing-Puente, PhD, "Parent Support,"
Cutting-Edge Therapies for Autism

507. Parent support groups, often led by a mental-health clinician, are provided regularly by many schools and local organizations. Such groups provide opportunities for parents to share their experiences, discuss ways of helping their children (e.g., by sharing information on treatment protocols and behavioral strategies), and caring for themselves. With the guidance of mental-health clinicians, parents can receive psychoeducation about the latest research on ASDs and treatment and strategies that can help their children and themselves.

—Lauren Tobing-Puente, PhD, "Parent Support,"
Cutting-Edge Therapies for Autism

508. Message boards and listservs for parents of children with ASDs have become very popular in recent years. The benefits of message boards and listservs include their convenience and accessibility, without the challenges of scheduling face-to-face support groups. This can be especially helpful for parents who live in remote areas. However, online technology does not afford the personal contact of support groups or provide the same opportunity to develop true relationships with other parents. Without consistent moderation by a clinician, it is difficult to ensure that the content is appropriate and factual.

—Lauren Tobing-Puente, PhD, "Parent Support,"
Cutting-Edge Therapies for Autism

509. A support system is crucial—and not just a family-and-friends system, but a group of people familiar with autism who might be able to help you out with the intricacies of the condition.

510. No one can do autism alone. Find friends—they are necessary for survival.

—Judith Chinitz, MS, MS, CNC, author of *We Band of Mothers*

CHAPTER 42

Siblings

511. Look for support groups that support not only parents, but also siblings. You should also consider counseling. Talk with your pediatrician and your health-care professional to establish whether counseling is necessary; if the autistic child receives most of a parent's attention, his siblings might feel left out.

—www.adviceaboutautism.com/treating-autism-at-home.html

512. Your child's best teacher is his sibling, so encourage them to be a friend. Remember, a sibling can take direct measures where a parent can't. Your child's sibling is also your opportunity to teach: Try actively rewarding the sibling for the behaviors you are trying to encourage in your spectrum child. For example: "Mary, I love it when you ask me for help," said within earshot of Joe, who never does.

—Lynette Louise, MS, Board certified in
Neurofeedback by BCIA, NTCB

513. Siblings should have their own safe place, out of the way when you need to settle down or focus on your child with autism who may be melting down. After things calm down, return to your typical child and help him or her understand what occurred.

514. Let siblings be kids too! Don't expect sibs to become part-time parents. They can help out, sure, but allow them to aid in their own way, playing with or showing how to play to the child with autism. Do not put a sib in the mode of babysitter.

515. When having a party, ask family members to help out. Organize a rotating team of adults, where each individual spends a half hour with the child, this allows parents and siblings to enjoy themselves, and the child doesn't have to be exposed to the chaos of the party.

516. Consider a sibling support group. If there aren't any in your area, there are books written for siblings of all ages.

517. It's important that the sibling has his own space; he can keep it locked so that he has a place to keep his belongings out of reach from his brother with autism. It's hard to harbor tender feelings toward a brother who is destroying your precious model airplanes or twirling your favorite items. Make sure the sibling has an autism-free zone to call his own—even if it is only a closet to store his personal belongings.

—Chantal Sicile-Kira, www.chantalsicile-kira.com

CHAPTER 43

Friends and Family

518. Sometimes we feel uncomfortable when a good friend or relative has a child with autism, because we don't know how to react or what to say. Here are some tips from *41 Things to Know About Autism* by Chantal Sicile-Kira (www.chantalsicile-kira.com):

- If you were good friends before the diagnosis and were in contact often, don't change. Your friend may not have the free time they had before to see you, but you can stay connected by phone or e-mail. Keep those lines of communication open.

- Stay connected by continuing to invite them over. If they can come, they'll come; if they can't, they won't. It can be hard for them to get out of the house, but don't give up, and keep the invitations coming.

- Find out a little bit about autism. Go to reputable websites and get some basic information.

- Learn more than you advise. It can be tempting to tell them everything you hear about autism in the news, but your friend has probably heard it all. Instead, offer an ear and some practical help.

- Is there some way you can help by offering them some precious time? They may not need advice, but they could sure use a break. Could you watch the child with autism for a few hours? Or maybe take the siblings out? How about dropping off a home-cooked meal one night?

- Don't ignore the child with autism because you don't know how to connect with him. Follow his lead and show interest in what he is doing. Show him something he might like. You can ask the parents for tips on how to interact with him; they will surely appreciate the overtures.

519. Convey helpful hints to others who will be interacting with your child. For example, suggest that they:

- Speak slowly and use simple language
- Use concrete terms
- Repeat simple questions
- Allow time for responses
- Give lots of praise
- Do not attempt to physically block self-stimulating behavior
- Remember that each individual with autism is unique and may act differently than others

520. The child or teen with autism may look like they are not paying attention, but they are taking in everything that is going on around them. They are listening to you even if they are not looking at you. Not being able to talk does not mean they don't understand you, or that they have nothing to communicate. Treat each child as if they understand what is being said in their presence. Give them the benefit of the doubt.

—Chantal Sicile-Kira, www.chantalsicile-kira.com

Examples for Family and Friends

Here are some everyday examples to help friends and family understand autism using familiar frameworks from "Parent Tips: Explaining Autism Using Everyday Examples" by Shelly McLaughlin, Pathfinders for Autism, 2009, www.pathfindersforautism.org:

521. Verbal does not mean smarter: Have you ever had a bad case of laryngitis? It was frustrating not being able to say what you meant or ask for things you needed, wasn't it? But while you couldn't speak, you were still processing information, and your intelligence level certainly didn't change. And were you given the benefit of alternative communication by using a pencil and paper, or a computer?

522. Running out of the classroom: Sensory overload might be difficult for most of us to appreciate. So imagine putting a desk inside the Harbor Tunnel during rush hour. About forty feet away from the desk stands a teacher who is going to orally give you algebraic word problems to complete. How long would you be able to sit there with the flashing lights and thunderous sounds of the cars racing by? And how well would you do on those algebra problems?

523. Let's continue with more on sensory issues. Have you ever had a tag in your shirt that really bothered you? Yes? Good. Now let's add cactus needles to that tag. Lots of them. We don't know why people with autism have incredibly heightened sensitivities, but they are very real.

524. Let's pretend you and your child are attending a birthday party where a magician is performing. Your child is jumping up and excitedly running over to the magician or calling out and another parent is noticeably annoyed and asks you to control your child. While we would all agree that this parent perhaps needs his own time-out, remind him how it feels when we go to a baseball or football game and our team has just hit a home run or scored a touchdown. We jump, we yell, we high-five the strangers behind us. If only the rest of us could experience that level of joy from everyday activities.

525. We have all experienced the joy of preparing our taxes. You were in that "tax zone"—your mind fully concentrating on receipts, expenses, and wondering what other exemptions you might have forgotten. How would you have reacted if while in this zone, someone came along and turned your computer off? Or how would you react if, during the Super Bowl, in a close game during the fourth quarter, your cable suddenly went out? That's how our child who is working on a puzzle feels when you suddenly announce it's time to pack up and go.

526. We've been in the elevator and have seen "that look" in our children's eyes, and we know what they are about to do. Yes—they are going to hit every button. As the other passengers begin to roll their eyes, ask them to take a moment (because you have the time now on this long elevator ride!) and think of freshly baked chocolate chip cookies. But they can't have one. The soft doughy centers, the gooey chocolate, the irresistible smell. And it's a giant plate full, so no one would even notice if one was missing. And the plate is so close it's almost touching their shirts. But, they are not allowed to eat one, and really, they need to pretend the cookies aren't there. How easy is that?

527. How often have you gotten an e-mail or sent an e-mail and the intention of the message was completely misunderstood? Without the verbal tones and facial cues most of us rely on for message interpretation, it's not uncommon to misread intent. Now, imagine all of your communication was carried out by tone-deaf e-mails, and you had to guess the intent of each message. Or, travel to a faraway country and try to understand metaphors that are culturally specific and make no sense to you. Think how much more comfortable you would be in that country if people just said exactly what they meant.

528. There is a book called *41 Things to Know about Autism,* by Chantal Sicile-Kira. You can give it to those who need to know more about autism—such as your relatives—so they can understand more about autism and its effects on the family. It explains very simply things such as the emotional and financial effects of autism on the family, why these kids and teens act the way they do, how you can help as a grandparent, what to do if you are a neighbor, how you can help as a friend, why sticking to diets and treatments are so important, and so on. It's an easy read.

CHAPTER 44

Home Help

529. As with most services, I have found the best sitters and helpers from other parents. You can also ask around at your son's school, camp, or play group. Many times some of the folks who work with the kids during the day are available to work at your home, either performing therapy or just supervising while you are out for a night of respite.

530. Check out your local colleges, which will usually post your sitter requests with the appropriate department, possibly in the special-needs education department.

The following tips for when you are organizing home help are adapted from the Indiana Resource Center for Autism at the Indiana Institute on Disability and Community at Indiana University, http://newsinfo.iu.edu/web/page/normal/6076.html.

531. Search out trustworthy caregivers. Government and public agencies can provide information about respite caregivers, usually through a Bureau of Developmental Disabilities or similar office. Teachers and friends familiar with respite services can also be good sources for references. Beverly Vicker, a speech pathologist with the Indiana Resource Center for Autism at Indiana University's Indiana Institute on Disability and Community, recommends the book, *A "Stranger" Among Us: Hiring In-Home Support for a Child with Autism Spectrum Disorder or Other Neurological Differences* by Lisa Lieberman, as an excellent resource for the hiring process.

532. Put yourself in their shoes. "The guiding directive for the entire endeavor of providing information for respite workers is to project yourself into the role of the respite worker," Vicker said. "What would you want to know in order to feel comfortable and confident to handle routine situations, as well as the unexpected ones that might occur in your household?" Putting this information in writing will reduce anxiety for both parents and care providers.

533. And then, on the side of over preparing: Although excessively detailed information might overwhelm caregivers in some situations, it is generally better to have written information on hand than to assume care providers have all the necessary background knowledge. "One cannot assume that the caregiver will remember all spoken instructions, particularly as a crisis arises," Vicker said.

534. Lastly, think ahead. Prepare your materials before the first day of respite services. "This way you are less likely to forget or overlook important information," Vicker said.

535. Once you hire someone, you want to keep them if they are good. Here are some tips on supervising people to work in your home with your son:

- Make sure the responsibilities are clear, including the times you are expecting them, and that they are responsible for communicating any changes to you as soon as possible.
- Have a calendar—in the kitchen or online—easily available where people can see special appointments or changes in scheduling.
- If you expect some degree of flexibility on their part, be prepared to be flexible for them.
- Make sure you have everything they need to do their work, and that everything has a specific place so things are easily found.
- Remember that they are there to help your child and not to be your counselor. Don't overburden them with all the problems you are having with, say, the school district.
- Remember to keep boundaries—keep your rapport with them respectful and professional.
- Have high expectations of their job performance, but make sure you have what they need to get the job done.

—Chantal Sicile-Kira, www.chantalsicile-kira.com

SECTION 7

....

Daily Life

L ittle strokes fell great oaks.

—Benjamin Franklin as Poor Richard

CHAPTER 45

Teaching Basic Skills

536. Begin teaching independence and daily living skills early on. It might take your child some time to perfect them. It's better to start earlier than later. Try things like having them set the table for dinner or preparing their own lunch.

—Megan Miller, Head Teacher

537. Get your child involved. Even if your child cannot complete the entire task, break down daily routines to give them a role. For example, give your child a shoelace to pull when untying laces, fasten the zipper and then allow your child to finish the task by pulling the zipper up, etc. Add more steps as your child's skills develop to further increase his/her independence.

—Jenn Gross, OTR/L

538. My son had trouble learning his right from his left. We discovered that he knew the sign (ASL) for R and the sign for L, so we gave him a visual hint with directional questions. In two days he got it without using the signs. Now he leads the pack, and we can tell him to go left or right to navigate places like the mall.

—Nancy Rannazzisi, Mom to Nicholas

539. In older nonverbal children and adults, touch is often their most reliable sense. It is often easier for them to feel. Letters can be taught by letting them feel plastic letters. They can learn their daily schedule by feeling objects a few minutes before a scheduled activity. For example, fifteen minutes before lunch, give the person a spoon to hold. Let them hold a toy car a few minutes before going in the car.

> —Temple Grandin, PhD, author of *Thinking in Pictures* and *The Way I See It*; www.autism.com/ind_teaching_tips.asp

540. Teaching generalization is often a problem for children with autism. To teach a child to generalize the principle of not running across the street, it must be taught in many different locations. If he is taught in only one location, the child will think that the rule only applies to one specific place.

> —Temple Grandin, PhD, author of *Thinking in Pictures* and *The Way I See It*; www.autism.com/ind_teaching_tips.asp

541.

Sequencing is very difficult for individuals with severe autism. Sometimes they do not understand when a task is presented as a series of steps. An occupational therapist successfully taught a nonverbal autistic child to use a playground slide by walking his body through climbing the ladder and going down the slide. It must be taught by touch and motor rather than showing him visually. Putting on shoes can be taught in a similar manner. The teacher should put her hands on top of the child's hands and move the child's hands over his foot so he feels and understands the shape of his foot. The next step is feeling the inside and the outside of a slip-on shoe. To put the shoe on, the teacher guides the child's hands to the shoe and, using the hand–over–hand method, slides the shoe onto the child's foot. This enables the child to feel the entire task of putting on his shoe.

—Temple Grandin, PhD, author of *Thinking in Pictures* and *The Way I See It*; www.autism.com/ind_teaching_tips.asp

Chapter 46

Improving Communication Skills

542. Our actual words carry far less meaning than nonverbal cues. The words themselves carry many meanings, depending on nonverbal cues. Ten compelling nonverbal forms of communication applicable to day-to-day communications are: vocal, facial, gestural, postural, proxemic, spatial, rhythm, movement, clothing and body decoration, and drawing.

—Ronald Mah, *Getting Beyond Bullying and Exclusion PreK–5*

543. Remember that behavior is communication. If a nonverbal child has no communication system, they will learn to communicate inappropriate behaviors. Often educators and parents are hesitant to use alternative systems of communications (i.e., PECS, typing, sign language) because they are afraid it will hinder speech developing, or that it is like giving up on their child or student. However, research has proven just the opposite: These alternative communication methods enhance the child's ability to speak.

—Chantal Sicile-Kira, www.chantalsicile-kira.com

544. Be careful not to put the individual's name at the beginning of each instructional cue. Gain his or her attention, pause, and then give the instructional cue. If we begin each instructional cue with a name, he might only attend to the name and not the content of the instructional cue. They might not attend to instructions given to a group by someone who is not speaking directly to him or her, and saying his or her name first.

—Barbara T. Doyle, MS, coauthor of *ASD from A to Z*

545. Use shorter sentences. Rule of thumb: Use sentences one to three words longer than the sentences your child uses. Note: This rule does not include Scripted Language, the little phrases your child understands that you say all the time in the exact same way.

—Tahirih Bushey MA-CCC, Autism Games, http://sites
.google.com/site/autismgames/home/parent-tips

546. Show your child what you mean. Children who have difficulty comprehending language often watch what others are doing very carefully—at least, when they are interested. If you are going to show your child something, you can say "Watch!" You should be saying "Just watch! I will show you" so often that your child tunes right in when you say this, and watches what you do next. Teach your child to watch when told to watch by doing very interesting things after you say it.

—Tahirih Bushey MA-CCC, Autism Games, http://sites
.google.com/site/autismgames/home/parent-tips

547. Make your own PECS. I took photos of my son's favorite foods, activities, and places. Using iPhoto or a similar program, you can arrange and order wallet-sized photos to place into a photo book or business-card holder for easy access at home and on the road.

548. You can also casually demonstrate the meaning of words as you talk about what you are doing. For example: "Here is juice. Mommy will pour juice. Just a little bit. Not too much. Oh! You want more. You can say 'More juice.' Mommy will pour just a little juice. More? You are thirsty! Mommy will pour a LOT!" This strategy is called Parallel Talk. It is where you talk about what you are doing as you do things. Remember the rule of thumb, though, and don't use sentences that are too long.

—Tahirih Bushey MA-CCC, Autism Games, http://sites .google.com/site/autismgames/home/parent-tips

549. Help your child shift attention between you and a toy. Children with autism often want to control the toys or other materials once they are engaged with something. Then, all their mental energy goes to that toy. You, their play-partner, are ignored! This makes it hard for you to build your child's communication and interaction skills. The goal is to create an activity in which you are an integral part of your child's play, and your child finds it easy (or at least worth the effort) to shift attention back and forth between you and the toy or the activity.

—Tahirih Bushey MA-CCC, Autism Games, http://sites .google.com/site/autismgames/home/parent-tips

550. Become the source of good things. Imagine your child wants to play an inset puzzle. You can sit beside your child and play with the puzzle, but your child is likely to ignore you. Worse, you might be perceived as human interference. He or she might get very agitated if you even touch the puzzle pieces. But if you have all the puzzle pieces and you find a creative way to give them to your child, then you are not interfering. Instead, you are providing what is needed in a most interesting manner.

—Tahirih Bushey MA-CCC, Autism Games, http://sites
.google.com/site/autismgames/home/parent-tips

551. Conversations occur when there is a need. If you have a collection of items that your child likes to choose from, you might want to make this collection visible but up on a shelf where it can't be independently retrieved. Put items in a bottle with a tightly shut lid. Even a clear plastic bag or clear plastic bottle will work, because this allows your child to see the desired item but not get it. I like Ziploc bags; at least some kids don't know how to get into them. You might need to clutch one end of the bag, though!

—Tahirih Bushey MA-CCC, Autism Games, http://sites
.google.com/site/autismgames/home/parent-tips

552. If you just hand over a snack item, there is no opportunity to discuss . . . anything! But put two different kinds of snacks in a clear bag, and you create an opportunity for discussion before your child eats.

553. When pursuing augmentative and alternative communication (AAC) solutions for a nonverbal child, it's important to remember that such solutions rarely work in isolation. Though universally associated with electronic speech-generating technology, AAC includes self-expressive strategies that we all use naturally, such as writing, gestures, and eye contact. Simple AAC tools—from picture symbol cards to digital photographs imported to a speech-generating device or organized in a scrapbook—can help keep communication predictable and meaningful for your child. Successful communication often happens when use of multiple modalities (including your child's verbal approximations) coincides with realistic expectations from typically speaking communication partners.

—Patti Murphy, Writer, DynaVox Mayer-Johnson

554. As a child develops communication skills, elements of predictability in dynamic speech-generating technology can reduce the stress of learning. Along with voice output that's easy to listen to, many devices offer built-in visual supports such as vocabulary that's color-coded by parts of speech. Words and phrases are readily identified by images (icons) with corresponding text on the display screen. Many devices also offer extensive preprogrammed vocabulary, sometimes organized by the child's age and cognitive ability level, keeping the technical requirements of parents and caregivers to a minimum.

—Patti Murphy, Writer, DynaVox Mayer-Johnson

555. Nonverbal children and adults will find it easier to associate words with pictures if they see the printed word and a picture on a flashcard. Some individuals do not understand line drawings, so it is recommended to work with real objects and photos first. The picture and the word must be on the *same* side of the card.

—Temple Grandin, PhD, author of *Thinking in Pictures* and *The Way I See It*; www.autism.com/ind_teaching_tips.asp

556. Some autistic individuals do not know that speech is used for communication. Language learning can be facilitated if language exercises promote communication. If the child asks for a cup, then give him a cup. If the child asks for a plate, when he wants a cup, give him a plate. The individual needs to learn that when he says words, concrete things happen. It is easier for an individual with autism to learn that their words are wrong if the incorrect word resulted in the incorrect object.

> —Temple Grandin, PhD, author of *Thinking in Pictures* and *The Way I See It*; www.autism.com/ind_teaching_tips.asp

557. Children who have difficulty understanding speech have a hard time differentiating between hard consonant sounds such as "D" in dog and "L" in log. My speech teacher helped me to learn to hear these sounds by stretching out and enunciating hard consonant sounds. Even though the child might have passed a pure-tone hearing test, he might still have difficulty hearing hard consonants. Children who talk in vowel sounds are not hearing consonants.

> —Temple Grandin, PhD, author of *Thinking in Pictures* and *The Way I See It*; www.autism.com/ind_teaching_tips.asp

558. Many people with autism are visual thinkers. I think in pictures. I do not think in language. All my thoughts are like videotapes running in my imagination. Pictures are my first language, and words are my second language. Nouns were the easiest words to learn because I could make a picture in my mind of the word.

—Temple Grandin, PhD, author of *Thinking in Pictures* and *The Way I See It*; www.autism.com/ind_teaching_tips.asp

559. Avoid long strings of verbal instructions. People with autism have problems with remembering the sequence. If the child can read, write the instructions down on a piece of paper. I am unable to remember sequences. If I ask for directions at a gas station, I can only remember three steps. Directions with more than three steps have to be written down. I also have difficulty remembering phone numbers because I cannot make a picture in my mind.

—Temple Grandin, PhD, author of *Thinking in Pictures* and *The Way I See It*; www.autism.com/ind_teaching_tips.asp

560. The four key language skills are: vocabulary, clarity of speech, sentence length, and conversational give-and-take. Show your child the power of his language by being responsive when he says something to you, especially if it's a new word or sentence.

—www.education.com/magazine/article/Ten_Tips_ for_Helping_Your

561. Some children and adults can sing better than they can speak. They might respond better if words and sentences are sung to them. Some children with extreme sound sensitivity will respond better if the teacher talks to them in a low whisper.

—Temple Grandin, PhD, author of *Thinking in Pictures* and *The Way I See It*; www.autism.com/ind_teaching_tips.asp

562. Eat as a family, preferably at the same time and eating the same food, and use that time for development of communication skills.

—Dr. Betty Jarusiewicz, "Neurofeedback (Neurotherapy or EEG Biofeedback)," *Cutting-Edge Therapies for Autism*

CHAPTER 47

Improving Social Skills

563. Children with autism do not naturally know how to ask for help, and this is a social skill that needs to be taught. For example, at recess, if a little child's shoelace becomes undone, the child will naturally go to ask the teacher for help in tying it up again. Not so the child with autism. You can teach this with children when they are requesting something they are having difficulty opening or reaching by pairing it with the spoken word or icon. Then, teaching them to come looking for you when they need help is the next step.

—Chantal Sicile-Kira, www.chantalsicile-kira.com

564. When your son is little, you can arrange playdates for him. As he gets older, you will have to teach him how to initiate contact with others, such as how to call and arrange to meet someone, how to send a text message, or leave a voice-mail message.

565. To prevent teenage boys from giving the wrong "signal," teach them that staring at certain parts of another's anatomy is rude and inappropriate. The rule should be that a person should never stare at the private parts of another person's body, the area normally covered by a bathing suit (male or female).

566. An ASD teen boy may not be able to "read" the cues from another person as to whether the interest is reciprocal. The teen needs to have explicit instruction about indications that someone likes them, as opposed to being interested romantically.

567. The "hidden curriculum"—the unstated rules in social situations—is something that needs to be taught to boys with autism, as they don't pick it up by osmosis like the other boys. As teens, it can become even more challenging. A good resource to help teach them what they need to know is *The Hidden Curriculum: Practical Solutions for Understanding Unstated Rules in Social Solutions* by Brenda Smith-Myles et al.

568. Teenage boys with autism may be physically maturing at the same rate as their teenage peers, but emotionally, they tend to mature much later. This creates problems sometimes in social situations at school, as the other boys start discussing dating and girls, something the boy with autism may not be interested in at that time.

569. Children with AS may be particularly prone to self-righteous vengeance because they often feel victimized for no reason they can discern. They may have done something or several things that have been disturbing or hurtful to others, but do not realize it due to misreading social cues from offended parties.

—Ronald Mah, *Getting Beyond Bullying and Exclusion PreK–5*

570. The 5-Point Scale of Touching and Talking illustrates the various degrees of interaction, and can help your child both understand and describe social interaction in a more concrete way:

(1) Thinking in a friendly way;

(2) Looking in a friendly way;

(3) Talking in a friendly way;

(4) Saying mean things;

(5) Punching/kicking.

—Brenda Smith Myles, *Children and Youth with Asperger's Syndrome*

Chapter 48
Improving Reading Skills

The following tips are adapted from "11 Tips to Encourage Reading in Children with Autism" by Alice Woolley, www.insidethebubble.co.uk.

571. Read daily and follow up. Try to get into the habit of some daily reading, because you want your child to remember what he learned the previous day, and to build on it.

572. Even a little daily reading does the trick. Don't put it all off until the weekend, and then attempt a marathon literacy session. It is far easier to concentrate for a short space of time, depending on the age of your child and his normal attention span. You might need to start at just five minutes at a time, increasing as your child gets older to around forty-five minutes; beyond that time, you will get less and less return for your efforts.

573. Use "cvc" (consonant-vowel-consonant) words first. Many books for children, even early board books and first readers, will not be designed with your child's vocabulary in mind. Some of them even include words that children at the earliest reading levels will not have a hope of being able to pronounce, such as "xylophone" or "through." Three-letter cvc words are among the easiest to pronounce. Ensure that any material you give your child early on has plenty of these.

574. Rhyme and repetition: *The Cat in the Hat* by Dr Seuss is a good book for beginners due to its repetition of "cvc" rhyming words. Repeated words are obviously easier to remember.

575. Start with words that are pronounced as they are spelled. Even some short words aren't pronounced phonetically; for example, words such as *what, was, two, girl, one,* and *are.* Avoid dealing with these words until your child is fairly confident with words that are pronounced the way they are written. When he is successfully reading words such as *cat, bin,* or *get,* gradually introduce words with more difficult pronunciations.

576. Persevere. Although it's not uncommon for children with autism to experience reading difficulties, it's also not unknown for an apparently hopeless situation to turn around as soon as they reach the right stage of development. Sometimes, things just click into place.

577. Don't let your child guess. Sometimes your child will take clues about what he is reading from the surrounding pictures. Also, if he is overly familiar with a story, he might simply remember how it goes without having to read. In order to assess his true reading level, you will sometimes need to use text, and to vary the stories frequently. Again, this is where a chalkboard or text-only flashcards will come in handy.

578. Words hold secrets. A good way of encouraging reluctant readers is to write down juicy secrets that he will want to uncover. Make it into a game for learning prepositions, or simply write down any interesting events or activities for that week. Keep it simple and short.

579. Shopping lists: As soon as he is able, encourage your child to read and write shopping lists.

580. Pictures: Picture books might have drawbacks for assessing a child's reading level, but good pictures will attract him to books in general, and introduce the idea of stories that exist only in the imagination.

581. Improve concentration. In order to get the best out of any reading session, your child should be as alert as possible. Don't confine reading to just before bedtime. Ideally take a short, brisk walk or some other form of mild exercise just before you start. Also, make sure your child has a drink of water (not soda or juice) beforehand, because dehydration impairs alertness.

582. Individuals with visual processing problems often find it easier to read if black print is printed on colored paper to reduce contrast. Try light tan, light blue, gray, or light green paper. Experiment with different colors. Avoid bright yellow—it might hurt the individual's eyes. Irlen colored glasses might also make reading easier.

> —Temple Grandin, PhD, author of *Thinking in Pictures* and
> *The Way I See It*; www.autism.com/ind_teaching_tips.asp

583. Some autistic children will learn reading more easily with phonics, and others will learn best by memorizing whole words. I learned with phonics. My mother taught me the phonics rules and then had me sound out my words. Children with lots of echolalia will often learn best if flashcards and picture books are used so that the whole words are associated with pictures. It is important to have the picture and the printed word on the same side of the card. When teaching nouns the child must hear you speak the word and view the picture and printed word simultaneously. An example of teaching a verb would be to hold a card that says "jump," and you would jump up and down while saying "jump."

> —Temple Grandin, PhD, author of *Thinking in Pictures* and
> *The Way I See It*; www.autism.com/ind_teaching_tips.asp

584. Several parents have informed me that using the closed captions on the television helped their child to learn to read. The child was able to read the captions and match the printed words with spoken speech. Recording a favorite program with captions on a tape would be helpful because the tape can be played over and over again and stopped.

—Temple Grandin, PhD, author of *Thinking in Pictures* and *The Way I See It*; www.autism.com/ind_teaching_tips.asp

CHAPTER 49

Improving Academic Skills

585. Many autistic children get fixated on one subject, such as trains or maps. The best way to deal with fixations is to use them to motivate schoolwork. If the child likes trains, then use trains to teach reading and math. Read a book about a train and do math problems with trains. For example, calculate how long it takes for a train to go between New York and Washington.

—Temple Grandin, PhD, author of *Thinking in Pictures* and *The Way I See It*; www.autism.com/ind_teaching_tips.asp

586. Adults [should] devise a learning activity in which the child can successfully participate within the time frame his threshold will permit. Once the child accomplishes the prescribed task(s), reward him with his favorite item or activity.

—Bill Moss, "Linwood Method," *Cutting-Edge Therapies for Autism*

587. Let children look for an object in warmed sand or discriminate between several objects in sand by touching. Exercise explorative touching, without eye contact, with two-dimensional shapes as a pre-exercise for visual exploration of letters and other forms.

—Bob Woodward and Dr. Marga Hogenboom, *Autism: A Holistic Approach*

588. Use concrete visual methods to teach number concepts. My parents gave me a math toy that helped me to learn numbers. It consisted of a set of blocks that had a different length and a different color for the numbers one through ten. With this I learned how to add and subtract. To learn fractions my teacher had a wooden apple that was cut up into four pieces and a wooden pear that was cut in half. From this I learned the concept of quarters and halves.

—Temple Grandin, PhD, author of *Thinking in Pictures* and *The Way I See It*; www.autism.com/ind_teaching_tips.asp

589. Some individuals with autism will respond better and have improved eye contact and speech if the teacher interacts with them while they are swinging on a swing or rolled up in a mat. Sensory input from swinging or pressure from the mat sometimes helps to improve speech. Swinging should always be done as a fun game. It must *never* be forced.

—Temple Grandin, PhD, author of *Thinking in Pictures* and *The Way I See It*; www.autism.com/ind_teaching_tips.asp

CHAPTER 50
Improving Handwriting Skills

590. Do the following regularly, and improvements in fine motor skills will be attained:

- Clay modeling
- Finger-painting
- Squeezing small balls or hand exercisers
- Lacing beads
- Weaving and tying activities
- Sorting small items into slots
- Winding up toys
- Piano play
- Finger puppet play
- Pouring activities (water, sand, etc.)

—Karen Plumley, "Improving Handwriting in Students with Autism," Suite101.com, www.suite101.com/profile.cfm/papaya42

591. Kids with autism might also struggle with pencil holding and pressure, grasping and pressing down too tightly and causing the writing utensil to break frequently, or gripping the pencil too loosely so that it wobbles. In either case, the student might benefit from weighted pencils, pencil grips, pencils with attached supportive elastic wristbands, and special no-slip paper.

—Karen Plumley, "Improving Handwriting in Students with Autism," Suite101.com, www.suite101.com/profile.cfm/papaya42

592. Adjust classroom handwriting requirements for autistic students. If a classroom writing assignment is long, a teacher might want to break it up into smaller sessions for the child with autism. Even better, have the child use a computer to type out larger writing projects instead of requiring him to write several pages.
—Karen Plumley, "Improving Handwriting in Students with Autism," Suite101.com, www.suite101.com/profile.cfm/papaya42

593. Author and clinical psychologist Tony Attwood stated in *The Complete Guide to Asperger's Syndrome* (Jessica Kingsley Publishers, 2007, pp. 263–265) that he believes handwriting is becoming an obsolete skill. Therefore, teaching typing and computer skills to students with autism might be a lesson that needs just as much attention as manual handwriting, if not more.
—Karen Plumley, "Improving Handwriting in Students with Autism," Suite101.com, www.suite101.com/profile.cfm/papaya42

594. I had the worst handwriting in my class. Many autistic children have problems with motor control in their hands. Neat handwriting is sometimes very hard. This can totally frustrate the child. To reduce frustration and help the child to enjoy writing, let him type on the computer. Typing is often much easier.

—Temple Grandin, PhD, author of *Thinking in Pictures* and *The Way I See It*; www.autism.com/ind_teaching_tips.asp

595. Check out the program Writing with Symbols. It's an easy-to-use typing program that actually talks as the words are typed. The program places pictures on each word written in a sentence.

—Pamela Downing, "Going Out into the Community with an Autistic Child," www.brownsvilleherald.com/articles /autistic-106258-child-community.html

CHAPTER 51

Homework Tips

Tips 596–599 are provided by Cathy Purple Cherry, AIA, LEED AP

Our 19 year old autistic son is on a certificate track, not a diploma track, at his school. Our focus now for his education is life skills and independence. He is at a 4th grade math level and 7th grade English level. My tips come from raising this autistic child.

596. Once our son got into middle school, I needed to figure out what I felt was important for his education and future. Don't look just to the day or year. As a parent of an autistic child, look far forward into their adulthood. This significantly impacts the educational decisions you make and the way you advocate during his or her school years.

597. Strong communication with your ASD child's teachers and special educational coordinator is pivotal. You should use email and document, document, document. Keep this correspondence as well as it may be needed for reference in future IEP meetings. My son was an A student but would only answer one of 10 questions on a sheet of paper. For me, it was important to have documentation from the teacher that he got his A's for effort only because I felt his grades misrepresented his processing abilities to the Board of Education.

598. Determine from your child's teachers how much time they want spent on homework. I got to the place where each teacher wrote at the top of their assignments the amount of time to be spent on the piece. I then sat my son down, set a timer, and when it went off, I stopped his efforts. It did not matter if he had only processed one question. Homework in an autistic child's world, in my opinion, is not nearly as important as him doing things he likes to do or doing things that help prepare him for independence. And more significantly, the sanity of the whole family is far more important than completing struggling homework.

599. Assess your child's academic gifts and work with these. Do not angst over making your child perform academically in an area of education that he or she is not good at. Know that time is the best teacher for these kids and that all things with them take more time. End of story. Do NOT do your child's homework believing you are helping him or her. This can give a false impression to his educational team and come back to haunt you in his IEP meetings.

600.

**Tips for Helping an ADHD with Homework
(also applies to children with ASDs)**

By Laura Wilson, adhdchildren.suite101.com/article.cfm/tips-for-helping-an-adhd-child-with-homework

- For a child to get his homework done, he will need an environment conducive to studying. First, make sure the student has all materials at hand. A child with ADHD who has to wander off to find an eraser will have a difficult time settling down to concentrate again. Second, figure out what noise level is helpful for the student. Some children work best in absolute silence. Others need some white noise like the whir of a fan in the background. Even some types of music can help a child's productivity. Parents will need to experiment with different options, and then stick with what works best.
- Now that the routine and environment are set, parents can add in some other variables to see if they help the child.
- Allow a child to stand if sitting makes him jittery. The ability to move around a bit might help him concentrate. Use a square of tape on the floor to make a box for his feet if he wanders too much.
- Provide textures to aid in productivity. Attach some adhesive Velcro strips (soft side) to the desk for the child to rub his hand on, or make some stress balls of balloons filled with flour, rice, or sugar for the child to play with while he's thinking.
- Certain scents aid in concentration. Experiment with basil, pine, peppermint, or citrus scents to see if any of these help.
- Keep the mouth busy. For some children, chewing gum or

snacking on something crunchy (like apples or crackers) can help productivity.

- Check on the child often, before he goes too far down the wrong road. It's frustrating to have to do a whole assignment over, but if a parent can see a problem before it goes on too long, it won't be such a big deal.

- Give rewards. As with many parenting challenges, rewarding exceptional effort or work will motivate the child to continue to do his best.

- A student with Attention Deficit Disorder can be successful and productive during homework time. Parents who help their child create a positive environment and routine will see great results when used in cooperation with helpful strategies.

- Allow breaks after a predetermined amount of time. For example, set a timer for fifteen minutes for a younger child, and allow him a five-minute break to stretch, run around, or play with a pet. His work time will be more productive in short segments.

601. If a child needs less one-on-one support, then a parent can establish a routine of where and when a child should complete their homework each day. Oftentimes, as many autistic students respond well to lists and visual organizers, parents can help foster success by providing their child with a daily academic checklist. This checklist can include tasks such as: complete homework, put all materials in the correct class folders, make sure materials for tomorrow are in my book bag, and so forth.

—Grace Chen, "5 Tips for Helping Your Autistic Child Excel in Public Schools," www.publicschoolreview.com/articles/88

602.
Bonus Homework Tips, adapted from Michael Connor, http://mugsy.org/connor2.htm

- Focus the child's attention before any communication, such as by using his name, or some other arranged signal.

- Use clear, simple requests or instructions, one at a time.

- Analyze tasks to ensure they are manageable and within the child's attention span.

- Always check understanding, and repeat/rephrase instructions as necessary.

- Practice newly acquired skills in different settings, in order to foster generalization.

- Use various means of presentation, such as visual, physical guidance, or peer modeling.

- Teach what "finished" means, and ensure that the child knows what to do upon the completion of a given task.

- Use simple and shared charts to record progress, and regularly use praise or more tangible rewards to mark good performance.

- Emphasize visual cues and signals as *aides-mémoires.*

- Specifically teach common similes and metaphors, to reduce over-literalness and demonstrate that words are not always to be taken at face value.

- Link work to the child's particular interests.

- Explore word-processing and computer-based schemes for literacy development.

- Gradually increase the complexity of reading material (and use books designed for slower readers but with a more "grown-up" content).

- Allow the child to avoid certain activities (such as sports and games) which he might not understand or like, and support the child in open-ended and group tasks.

- Allow some access to obsessive behavior as a reward for positive efforts on tasks set.

- Remove or minimize distracters, or provide access to an individual work area, when a task requiring concentration is set.

Chapter 52

Managing Your Child's Environment

603. People on the autism spectrum are especially sensitive to sensory conditions such as sound, lighting, physical touch, and so on. Consider changes that might make your child more comfortable.
—Harold L. Doherty, "Tips for Securing a Teachers Assistant for Your Autistic Student," www.wellsphere.com/autism-autism
-spectrum-article/ta-tips-tips-for-securing-a-teachers-
assistant-for-your-autistic-student/146550

604. If your child has meltdowns or sensory issues when in a particular place (a specific playground or room), avoid that location for a period of two weeks, and then reintroduce it. This will provide a clue as to what is causing the trouble. For example, a particular playground might be too noisy or crowded for him to handle at this time.

605. Become an expert on your child. Figure out what triggers your kid's "bad" or disruptive behaviors and what elicits a positive response. What does your autistic child find stressful? Calming? Uncomfortable? Enjoyable? If you understand what affects your child, you'll be better at troubleshooting problems and preventing situations that cause difficulties.
—Reprinted with permission from Helpguide.org. See www.helpguide.org/mental/autism_help.htm for additional resources and support.

606. Observe your son's behavior and mood following meals, environment changes (going outside during the summer), and exposure to different lighting, sounds, and sights. Become Sherlock Holmes to pinpoint situations that need adjusting.

607. If a child covers his ears playfully, ask if he likes loud sounds muffled through his hands, or quiet like a whisper. Then act out the question. Get the child to indicate a preference and then thank him for helping you to do what makes him most comfortable. Now play with it! Tell him you like it sung and sing about your love for him. The idea is to desensitize and educate the sensory system while watching your child's cues and then teaching him to put words to his desires. Running from his actions as if you have hurt him with your exuberance will make it so.

—Lynette Louise, MS, Board certified in Neurofeedback by BCIA, NTCB

608. Keep a calm home environment and a good family atmosphere. An overstressed home will not allow a child with autism—who may have ADD, ADHD, and/or sensory processing issues—the secure and tranquil atmosphere he needs. Parents should try to create a harmonious and democratic family atmosphere. If the parents don't get along very well, the child will feel the tension.

609. Create a home safety zone. Carve out a private space in your home where your child can relax, feel secure, and be safe. This will involve organizing and setting boundaries in ways your child can understand. Visual cues can be helpful (colored tape marking areas that are off-limits, labeling items in the house with pictures). You might also need to safety-proof the house, particularly if your child is prone to tantrums or other self-injurious behaviors.

—Reprinted with permission from Helpguide.org. See www.helpguide.org/mental/autism_help.htm for additional resources and support.

610. Don't be afraid to discipline your child when necessary. It is important not to underestimate your child. Children with autism are capable of willful misbehavior. It can be a challenge to determine what is willful and what is not, but parents should not assume that all behaviors are unintentional. Much like a typical child, an autistic child can and should be told what he should or should not do.

CHAPTER 53

Family Activities

611. Parent–child activities for children with autism can include sports as well. Though autistic individuals often shy away from competitive team sports, parents can provide a relaxed atmosphere for tossing a football back and forth, learning to swing a golf club, or kicking a soccer ball into a net. These activities are useful for promoting motor coordination, which is an issue for many children with autism.

> —Angie Geisler, "Fun Activity Suggestions for Parents of Children with Autism," www.brighthub.com/education /special/articles/57559.aspx#ixzz0l0QC6jNt

612. Board games are fun for autistic children to play with parents and siblings. These children often gravitate toward games that involve logical and strategic thinking, such as memory games or puzzles. This type of activity allows the child to interact closely with family members.

> —Angie Geisler, "Fun Activity Suggestions for Parents of Children with Autism," www.brighthub.com/education /special/articles/57559.aspx#ixzz0l0QC6jNt

613. When parents of children with autism regularly plan cooperative activities, they help to increase a child's confidence level and to foster the communication skills that are necessary for participation in activities with both autistic and neurotypical peers.

—Angie Geisler, "Fun Activity Suggestions for Parents of Children with Autism," www.brighthub.com/education /special/articles/57559.aspx#ixzz0l0QC6jNt

614. Parent-child activities for children with autism can be conducted in either a one-on-one format or in conjunction with a larger group of families. These activity suggestions can be tailored to an autistic child's interests, strengths, and ability to communicate and follow instructions.

—Chantal Sicile-Kira, www.chantalsicile-kira.com

615. Activities that focus on sensory exploration, particularly those that involve visual and tactile learning, can easily be organized in the home environment. Some sensory activities that children with autism respond well to include finger-painting, water-table play, matching color flashcards, building block structures, and using Play-Doh (not for children on a gluten-free diet). Parents can bond with their child and encourage two-way communication by actively participating in these activities rather than allowing the child to play alone.

—Angie Geisler, "Fun Activity Suggestions for Parents of Children with Autism," www.brighthub.com/education /special/articles/57559.aspx#ixzz0l0QC6jNt

CHAPTER 54

Showing Affection

616. Never underestimate the power of a hug. Bear hugs show affection while giving your child input that helps them learn about their bodies to build better body awareness. This input is grounding and calming. Remember, light touch tends to be aversive, so when giving hugs, placing your hand on a shoulder, or rubbing your child's back, deep, firm pressure is the way to go, as long as it is safe. Don't be surprised if your child starts asking for more "hugs," "squeezes," and "rubs." If he resists hugs, talk to the OT about other ways to provide this input.

—Jenn Gross, OTR/L

617. Anyone who knows Temple Grandin *(Thinking in Pictures, Animals in Translation)* can attest to the fact that over the years, she has learned to show affection. She could not do so as a child, but if you saw the Emmy Awards show in August 2010, you will remember the long and close hugs she gave onstage to the producers of the HBO movie about her life. Temple is proof that the window of opportunity never closes, and that even if your daughter is not able to show affection to you right now, she can learn over time.

—Chantal Sicile-Kira, www.chantalsicile-kira.com

Showing Affection to Your Child with Sensory-Processing Issues

Tips by Cathy Purple Cherry, AIA, LEED AP

618. Affection can be shown to all people through words and imagery, not just through touch. Thus, surround your sensitive child with words and images of love.

619. Understand the sensory issues of your ASD child to avoid using or wearing materials that trigger a negative response. This may allow you to have successful physical contact.

620 Try approaching your child from various levels—maybe not standing full height but on your knees. You may find the point of initial touch changes the ASD child's response. You can even try lying down with your child before touching him. Also try various body areas for successful touch using different kinds of pressure. It may be that simple pressure to the top of the head where hair provides a layer of insulation is the best touch.

621 It may be difficult to accept that you cannot snuggle up to your autistic son or that he does not appear to be bonding with you. Work on accepting this fact yourself so that you do not go through your child's life feeling rejected. He did not ask to be born with these challenges.

622 When physical affection isn't an option, try the following:

- Use music and dance to show love as long as auditory processing sensitivities do not exist.
- Give something yummy to eat to show that you love him, and decorate it regardless of what it is. Remember the small things that reminded you your mother loved you. A peanut butter and jelly sandwich cut with heart-shaped cookies cutters is a good thing.

Bonus Tip: As you work to build levels of affection with your ASD child and get comfortable with the strategies above (or any that you create on your own) that work, do not neglect to inform caregivers and other family members about what you are doing. One weekend with the grandparents who may not be on the same page could cause a regression and undermine all your hard work.

CHAPTER 55

Eye Contact

623. While it is a goal to improve your child's eye contact, know that even though they may not look directly at you they can still be paying attention. Kids might sideways-look for social reasons (shyness), but some may also have visual issues (check with your doc), and it is possible that by angling their gaze away they are actually seeing you head-on. In light of this, encourage eye contact but do not punish for not receiving it.

624. Something you can do to improve eye contact is to be consistent in asking your son to look at your face whenever he wants something. You may not get it every time, but keep to it and respond quicker when he gives you eye contact. He will notice this and work to improve.

625. More on eye contact: When he asks for an object, hold it directly in front of your face and request eye contact. When he looks to retrieve the object use affect to reward his glance and make a game of it. Again, consistency is key; keep to it and he will make progress.

626. Autistic children learn a lot in situations in which they are not confronted. Take this into account. Autistic children notice more than you might first assume. Speak softly, and not always from the front but also from behind, for the autistic child is not yet self-assured when confronted by someone.

—Bob Woodward and Dr. Marga Hogenboom,
Autism: A Holistic Approach

CHAPTER 56

Teaching Behavioral and "Social" Management

627. Social Skills Tips from Michael Connor,
www.mugsy.org/connor2.htm

- Recognize that a change in manner or behavior may reflect anxiety or stress, which may be triggered by even a minor change in routine.
- Don't take apparently rude or aggressive behavior personally; recognize that the target for the child's anger may be unrelated to the source of that anger.
- Teach specific social rules/skills, such as turn-taking and social distance. You can also teach your child opening gambits for initiating and maintaining conversation. Enhance verbal expression (intonation) via drama, role-play, and audio- or videotaped feedback. This kind of intervention, with individual debriefing afterwards, may be particularly relevant for high school students.
- Specific teaching, via photographs or video recordings, of how feelings are expressed and communicated (and therefore recognized) can be very helpful.
- Protect the child from teasing during free times, and provide peers with some insight into the needs of children on the autistic spectrum.
- Provide regular opportunities for simple conversation, with increasing use of "how" and "why" questions.
- Use charts to record behavioral progress and as a basis for reinforcement.
- It's important to have enhanced supervision during practical or physical activities.

628. Make use of self-stimulating behaviors. While stimming is typically performed to gain a sensory escape or satisfy a physical need, if you join in during these periods you may gain a quick glance or other feedback and have the beginning of a communication to build on.

629. If your son is melting down or very upset, try to remain in a calm state and keep a steady, serene appearance. In many cases this can serve to calm him quicker than is typical.

630. If your child is hyperactive and out of control, don't be tempted to react by shouting to get him to stop; in an overcrowded or noisy location (playground, store), it is likely that the environment is overstimulating him to begin with, and shouting will only make things worse. Likewise, a sensation-craving kid might grab items off a store shelf or run around because the environment is so tempting and overwhelming to his regulatory ability. Scolding will only add to the turmoil and lead to feelings of guilt (by both) later on. To calm the child and get him regulated, remove him from the location, and use a soothing activity . . . Always remember to counterbalance a child's loss of control with calm words and gestures, and help the child reorganize and regain focus and attention.

—Stanley Greenspan, MD, *Overcoming ADHD*

631. Alternatively, the child might need you to be completely quiet.

632. Listen to your child's body language: Is he running, jumping, crashing onto the floor or into the wall? Does he prefer sedentary activities? Talk to your child's occupational therapist about the movements and sensations that your child seeks. Ask for a sensory diet to give your child consistent input and help satisfy these "cravings."

—Jenn Gross, OTR/L

633. Put your child to work. Heavy work that includes resistive activities (such as pushing, pulling, and carrying) provides input that is organizing and calming. At home you can have your child help with everyday chores while providing this important information to the body. Examples: pushing in chairs after mealtimes, pushing shopping carts at the grocery store, carrying heavier food items (rice, cans, etc.) and helping to put them away, carrying boxes of games to clean up, pulling the laundry basket to the machine, etc.

—Jenn Gross, OTR/L

634. We use our mouths to help us stay regulated and calm (think gum, sucking candies, biting your lip, or chewing the inside of your cheek). Give your child oral input by using straws to drink thick shakes, yogurt, applesauce, pudding, etc. Cut straws shorter if it is too difficult. Use narrower or longer straws to increase the challenge. Provide chewy (e.g., dried fruit) and crunchy foods (e.g., apples). This facilitates oral motor development while providing heavy work for the mouth. Talk to your child's speech or occupational therapist about other ways to provide oral input.

—Jenn Gross, OTR/L

635. Allow your son/daughter a significant amount of time to process and think after asking them a question. Thinking is hard work, but crucial for their development.

—Megan Miller, Head Teacher

CHAPTER 57

Computer Time

636. Apps! Apps run on the iPhone, iTouch, and iPad providing a range of choices for your son. There are literally hundreds of autism related apps, just search for autism in the app store. Some favorites include: Proloquo2Go™ (full-featured communication solution), Is that Gluten Free?, Learn to Talk, iPrompts®, ABA Flash Cards, and iMean (which turns the entire screen into a large-button keyboard with text display).

Bonus Tip: For a blog that reviews autism-related apps, check out Autism Epicenter: autismepicenter.net/blog/blog2.php/2010/06/01/autism-apps-that-will-help-you

637. Choose when your child will use the computer intentionally, and, just like television, sparingly. The computer has the potential to be wonderfully educational and the potential to be terribly harmful to your child's social development.
—Tahirih Bushey MA-CCC, Autism Games, http://sites
.google.com/site/autismgames/home/parent-tips

638. Use the computer as a social motivator rather than a break from social interaction. This means finding ways to interact with your child or help your child interact with others while using the computer, and insisting that the computer be used as a social tool.

—Tahirih Bushey MA-CCC, Autism Games, http://sites
.google.com/site/autismgames/home/parent-tips

639. Children and adults with visual processing problems can see flicker on TV-type computer monitors. They can sometimes see better on laptops and flat-panel displays, which have less flicker.

—Temple Grandin, PhD, author of *Thinking in Pictures* and
The Way I See It; www.autism.com/ind_teaching_tips.asp

640. Some children and adults with autism will learn more easily if the computer keyboard is placed close to the screen. This enables the individual to simultaneously see the keyboard and screen. Some individuals have difficulty remembering if they have to look up after they have hit a key on the keyboard.

—Temple Grandin, PhD, author of *Thinking in Pictures* and
The Way I See It; www.autism.com/ind_teaching_tips.asp

641. Many individuals with autism have difficulty using a computer mouse. Try a roller ball (or tracking ball) pointing device that has a separate button for clicking. Autistics with motor control problems in their hands find it very difficult to hold the mouse still during clicking.

> —Temple Grandin, PhD, author of *Thinking in Pictures* and *The Way I See It*; www.autism.com/ind_teaching_tips.asp

642. Some autistic individuals do not understand that a computer mouse moves the arrow on the screen. They might learn more easily if a paper arrow that looks *exactly* like the arrow on the screen is taped to the mouse.

> —Temple Grandin, PhD, author of *Thinking in Pictures* and *The Way I See It*; www.autism.com/ind_teaching_tips.asp

643. Help your child use new knowledge or skills learned on the computer in other places and in social situations. For example, if your child is playing a Dora the Explorer computer game in which Dora is finding treasures, and Swiper tries to steal treasures periodically, then make up a game in which you find the same treasures with your child around the house. Don't skip this step; take the time to figure out how to do this generalization step for every new computer game you introduce to your child, if possible. It is the tendency of children with ASD to learn in a fragmented way, and not to make the connections between things learned in one setting to things learned in another setting. The computer can become like an alternative world, but the skills learned on the computer should become useful in the real world.

—Tahirih Bushey MA-CCC, Autism Games, http://sites
.google.com/site/autismgames/home/parent-tips

644. Don't let your child play games that increase aggressive behavior. This is as destructive as watching videos that increase aggressive behavior. Many families have to eventually give up (or put away for several years) an expensive game system that they might have purchased with loving intentions, because the games on that system cause behavior problems. A child with ASD, by definition, has an uneven developmental profile, meaning the child is more mature in one area than in another. Many children with ASD are far less mature emotionally than intellectually. Use your judgment, not your child's age, as your guide to which computer activities are educational and appropriate.

—Tahirih Bushey MA-CCC, Autism Games, http://sites
.google.com/site/autismgames/home/parent-tips

645.

Beware that your resolve to limit computer use might weaken if you are not careful! Yes, the computer can teach your child new skills. And yes, your child might really enjoy time on the computer . . . but I have watched many parents struggle with a child who is addicted to the computer as though it were a drug. I have seen children who are willing to do violence to get more time on the computer. Uncontrolled use of the computer has a family-destroying potential similar to letting your child watch too many videos, or letting your child demand that you buy things whenever you shop, or letting your child's demands convince you to make him or her something different for dinner. There are certain predictable child demands that, if you give in to them, can make your family life very difficult and do more harm than good for your child. Uncontrolled computer use is one of these.

—Tahirih Bushey MA-CCC, Autism Games, http://sites
.google.com/site/autismgames/home/parent-tips

646. The computer is a wonderful tool for us all, and many of us love our computers inordinately, but we all have to learn to use them moderately and wisely. It is easier to be proactive on this than make a change in family rules, but, if need be, put the computer away for a while and start over with new rules a few months later.
—Tahirih Bushey MA-CCC, Autism Games, http://sites
.google.com/site/autismgames/home/parent-tips

647. Temple Grandin often says that letting your child or teen spend too much time on the computer without a purpose is not a good idea. You do want to encourage computer skills to develop, as they may lead to job or career possibilities. To do that, Temple suggests finding a mentor to come over once a week to teach different computer applications and develop skill areas that could be helpful for future employment.
—Chantal Sicile-Kira, www.chantalsicile-kira.com

CHAPTER 58

What You Have All Been Waiting for . . . Sleep Tips!

648. Sleep rules! Remember kids and parents perform better and will be happier with a good night's sleep. Do not allow medications or other treatments to limit this important function. Try melatonin if there are difficulties; it works for many kids on the spectrum and good for parents having trouble sleeping as well.

649. Chronic problems can occur in the absence of a consistent bedtime routine, which should include a specific bedtime and a clearly defined sleep location, both a bedroom and a bed.
—Ellen Notbohm and Veronica Zysk, *1001 Great Ideas for Teaching and Raising Children with Autism Spectrum Disorders*

650. Occasional sleep problems can result from many different sources and be difficult to analyze. Look at the possible side effects of any new medications, any change in diet, the need for a bowel movement, adjustments to schedule, or perhaps nap during the day. Once again a log of daily activities can help pinpoint the cause.

651. Blackout shades are a good option, and they have the added bonus of making bedrooms dark for deeper sleep during naps.

—Candi Summers, Autism & Parenting Examiner,
Examiner.com, http://exm.nr/9SfVh8

Sleeping tips from Cathy Purple Cherry, AIA, LEED AP

652. Our son is now 19. He was adopted from Russia at 3. He still rocks himself to sleep with a side to side motion. This motion is very soothing for him so we allow it to happen for a limited period of time. I have discovered that if I tell him to roll to his stomach, the rocking stops and he falls asleep faster. If you wonder why I limit the time, it is because he also goes to camp and school and has roommates. This motion and sound can be very frustrating to others. Thus, I teach them also to tell him to roll to his stomach after a few soothing minutes.

653. Recognize that even typically-developing children and mostly autistic children can't go from 60 mph to 0 mph in a short time limit. Thus, don't fool yourself to think you can just say, "Okay everyone. It's time for bed!" The time process related to preparing an autistic child for bed can be extensive due to the number of prompts required to take all the steps. Also, calm the house down well in advance of when you want to start the process by dimming or turning off lights and lowering noise levels from the TV or other children. For our family, I would say it took originally 2 hours for this process. Now, at his age of 19, I would say it takes a minimum of 30 minutes, but you must be firm in your voice tone to constantly move the child forward.

654. If the bedtime routine seems unending, speak with your pediatrician and psychiatrist about Melatonin, a naturally occurring compound found in plants and animals. It seems that when this pill is taken, within about 1 hour, you are definitely ready to fall asleep. A psychologist and pediatrician recommended this for our family. Be sure to check with your medical professional first for any interaction or issues.

655. When travelling with your whole family and staying at hotels, bedtime can be a nightmare. If you can, get two separate rooms—one for you and your autistic child and one for the rest of the family. This is smart and necessary planning.

656. What works for each ASD child can be different. Try tucking the blankets tightly around the child or allow the child to sleep in his or her clothes. Watch carefully for what seems to be patterns and obsessions and work with or through these. Do not try to make the child comply with your definition of proper bedtime routines.

657. A body pillow or even a sleeping bag can fill in for you when it's time for you child to make the transition to sleeping on his own. If your son is resistant to sleeping without you, try placing such an item in the bed with him to take up the extra space.

658. You can create a hotel-room setup: Trade your king or queen bed for a couple of twins, and put a table in between to build sleeping independence. Once they are comfortable with this, you can begin to move him to his own room. The next step in this process would be to let him fall asleep in his own room, with you, and then you can move to your own bed after he falls asleep.

659. Epsom salt baths. Give in the evening, and morning if time permits. Epsom salt promotes calming and acts as a mild chelator, pulling toxins from the body. It also promotes sleep.

660. Melatonin. Use at night, start with 1 mg, increase the dose as needed and as weight increases. Use the slow-release formulation for night awakenings, standard formulation for trouble falling asleep. This supplement is very safe and easy to go on and off in comparison to sleep drugs. Side benefits include more mellow days (a good night's sleep does wonders) and antioxidant properties.

CHAPTER 59

Organization

Tips in this chapter are adapted from "4 Tips For Helping Organize Children On The Autistic Spectrums Toys, Schedules And Schoolwork" by Heidi DeCoux, www.articleonlinedirectory.com/Art/470333/240/4-tips-for-helping-organize-children-on-the-autistic-spectrums-toys-schedules-and-schoolwork.html.

661. Create a bin system for your child's supplies and toys. Separate the types of toys and supplies into individual bins. Take photographs of each type of toy or supply contained within and tape the photograph to the front of each corresponding bin.

662. Display children's toys, supplies, and clothing. It is easier for autistic children to stay organized and function if they can see all of their belongings. Drawers do not usually work well for children on the autism spectrum. Hang as many of their clothes as possible, or fold them and place them on shelves, preferably cubbies. Place jeans in one cubby, sweatshirts in another, and so on. Socks, underwear, and pajamas are best placed in transparent bins with photographs taped to the front. If you don't have cubbies, you may tape photographs on the front of each drawer. If possible, do not combine items into one drawer.

663. Set up daily routines and stick to them as much as possible. Creating regular daily routines can make transitioning from one activity to another less upsetting. Children on the autism spectrum often thrive when they have daily routines and usually react poorly to changes in routines. Once a solid routine is created, small changes can be introduced slowly, and can help your child develop coping strategies to deal with transitions. It is best to introduce changes in routines in very small steps. Gradually, your child will be able to use strategies like social stories and self-talk to work through the anxiety they experience when making transitions.

664. An example of an organizing routine is to give your child a ten-minute heads-up before dinner each evening, and then have them set an egg timer for ten minutes. Teach them that when the timer goes off, they are to pick up all of their toys and place them in the appropriate bins. This establishes a routine, lets them know what to expect, gives them a ten-minute lead time, and then provides them with a distinct audio clue when it's time to pick up and get organized. It is important to have them set the egg timer, not you. It gets them more involved in the process so they will be more likely to follow through with the routine.

665. An addition to this routine could be that when the egg timer goes off and it's time to pick up and get organized, you could play a specific song that your child would come to recognize as the "pick up and get organized" song. This can make it fun, playful, and soothing, and can also help keep them on task so they will get the work done faster.

666. Create a visual schedule for your child. Picture schedules work best for autistic kids. Set up the picture schedule so that when your child is finished with the task/activity, they can move that picture to the "all-done" side. Essentially, you are creating an interactive picture schedule that your child can "control." Their picture schedule could also be organized by first, next, last. It will give them the order of tasks, and, once completed, they can move the picture to the "completed" side.

CHAPTER 60

Extreme Makeover: Home Edition for Autism

The following tips are adapted from *Autistic Spectrum Disorders: Understanding the Diagnosis & Getting Help by Mitzi Waltz*. Published by O'Reilly Media, Inc. Copyright © 2002 Mitzi Waltz. All rights reserved. Used with permission. http://oreilly.com/medical/autism/news/tips_life.html

The homes of most young children with autistic spectrum disorders have a certain uniformity. After a few incidents of shattered heirlooms and leaning towers of furniture, accessible areas tend to get a makeover in the direction of a simple, stripped-down look. Baby gates, locked doors, childproofing devices, and the like abound.

667. When shopping for new furniture, pay extra attention to sturdy, easy-to-clean pieces. You might want to use sticky-back Velcro or foam to secure a few knickknacks, but it's best to relegate the family china and precious ornaments to an inaccessible room or a locked (and hard to overturn or shake) china cabinet.

668. Bunk beds and other furnishings that invite acrobatics may not be a good idea for your child. Then again, they might, if your child tends to be unresponsive to her environment, but gets excited about climbing up to an upper bunk or bouncing on a springy mattress.

669. Likewise, shelves that could be used as steps up to precipitous locations should be removed, or very securely anchored.

670. Some children seem to have a compulsion to move furniture around, often using it to build ramps up to places they shouldn't be. Solutions include:

- Removing wheels or plastic sliders from furniture legs
- Choosing very heavy furnishings
- Weighting or blocking the movement of furniture with heavy concrete blocks hidden beneath stuffed couches and chairs
- Literally attaching furniture to walls or the floor with hook-and-eye fasteners or other hardware

671. For the early years, at least, it's good if you can learn to appreciate thrift-store chic. You'll feel a lot worse if your child picks holes in a $1,000 couch than if he damages a $75 sofa from a garage sale. Slipcovers are a good idea for protecting nice fabrics.

672. If you want to have one or more nice rooms, either lock them or be prepared to stand guard at all times. Experienced parents can attest that the latter option is not worth it—you definitely have better things to do with your days than worrying about stains on your Persian rugs. There will probably be a time when you can enjoy some of the finer things again, but now may not be that time.

Living with Your Autistic Child in Your Home
Tips by Cathy Purple Cherry, AIA, LEED AP

When an autistic child has siblings, especially younger ones, there can be considerable conflict that occurs in a home environment. There are simple practical design solutions and strategies that can be applied to your home to help reduce this conflict.

If you are designing a home from scratch, aside from implementing ADA strategies such as wider door openings, ramps, and ADA-approved light and plumbing fixtures for possible physical challenges your child may have, the following design items should be considered for the autism spectrum:

673. Increase the floor area between the kitchen counter and the kitchen island to a minimum of five to six feet. This helps improve the personal space of the family members and reduce the potential for touching and a sense of invasion.

674. If the house is a larger scale, include two staircases with each staircase a minimum of four feet in width to help reduce the possibility of path crossing.

675. Provide an en suite bathroom to the autistic child's bedroom. This eliminates the gross-out factor that can happen between two siblings, which is further amplified by the inappropriate judgment of the ASD child and the inappropriate reactions of the sibling.

676. Install an electric oven. Do not install gas. Curiosity with fire can be an issue with ASD children and teens, and this helps eliminate the risk of feeding that curiosity.

677. Use wood flooring, not carpet, so that you can hear the footsteps of the child or teen and understand their movements in your home. This gives you as a parent a chance to prevent conflict and poor judgment.

678. Install wood blocking behind drywall for all towel and robe hooks. The toggle bolts do not hold up to the strength of these individuals and their misjudgment in removing items from these hooks as they get older.

679. Install plywood behind the drywall and hallway areas or in their room to help prevent damage to the walls as oppositional behaviors develop during adolescence.

680. Overall, remember impulsivity leads to inappropriate decisions and conflict. The best strategy is "out of sight, out of mind." I learned this after our ASD son pulled a knife from a knife block visible on the kitchen counter and used it as a weapon to threaten someone at the age of ten. If you do not want my son to touch, steal, impulsively take or break something, then you must keep things out of sight. Keep all knives in a cabinet, all lighters hidden, all tools in a closet or in a secured area, all firearms and firecrackers in safes, and all money locked away.

If your home already exists, the following ideas can still be implemented:

681. Create a separate snack cabinet in the kitchen to prevent the siblings from being grossed out by the touching of shared food. When siblings are young, they have not yet developed the ability to respond appropriately to their autistic sibling. As is true in our home, this situation is compounded when the siblings are younger than the ASD teen.

682. Clearly define the outdoor play area for the ASD child. This area can be demarcated by plantings, structures, or sculptures. Defining this area allows the individual with special needs to do anything they desire without conflict with the other siblings also playing in the same yard.

683. Provide a preset number of drawers in the child's room for hoarded objects. Explain that if the drawers get filled, the child must remove objects to make more room for other items.

684. Completely eliminate the door locks specifically on the ASD child's bathroom, as well as bedroom. Our son likes to lock himself in the bathroom when he is having a fit. He is also known to stand outside his shower and pretend to bathe by wetting his hair. Without the lock, this allows me to knock on the door and then enter and check to see what he is doing.

685. Place timers in the ASD child's bedroom, bathroom, and the kitchen. Using timers aids in giving the individual a better sense of how long something should take. Matthew has no sense of time whatsoever. We started using these in his bathroom, as his showers were forty minutes long. These timers aided in Matthew learning better judgment as to how long something should take. We no longer use them, but do still at times need to prompt him or count down.

686. Place locks on certain cabinets to help control access to items that present dangers. Further, there may be obsessions with specific food items that need to be managed by placing these foods in these cabinets.

687. If necessary, set up the autistic teen's room like a college dormitory, providing relative independence from the rest of the house. As our son has gotten older, his strength has increased but his judgment has not improved. For the safety of our other children who are younger and smaller, it is necessary to strategize how to reduce the overlapping paths of our kids. We have discussed this strategy, as mealtime is definitely one of the worst times in our home due to the table manners, voice tone, poor reactions, and inappropriate behaviors of our ASD son.

SECTION 8

Productive Approaches to Parenting

If I had my child to raise over again,
I'd build self-esteem first, and the house later.
I'd finger-paint more, and point the finger less.
I'd do less correcting and more connecting.
I'd take my eyes off my watch, and watch with my eyes.
I'd take more hikes and fly more kites.
I'd stop playing serious, and seriously play.
I'd run through more fields and gaze at more stars.
I'd do more hugging and less tugging.
    —Diana Loomans, from "If I Had My Child to Raise Over Again"

Parenting; it's not just a job, it's an adventure!

    —Author unknown

CHAPTER 61

All the Time

688. Be consistent. Autistic children have a hard time adapting what they've learned in one setting (such as the therapist's office or school) to others, including the home. For example, your child might use sign language at school to communicate, but never think to do so at home. Creating consistency in your child's environment is the best way to reinforce learning. Find out what your child's therapists are doing and continue their techniques at home. It's also important to be consistent in the way you interact with your child and deal with challenging behaviors.

—Reprinted with permission from Helpguide.org. See www.helpguide.org/mental/autism_help.htm for additional resources and support.

689. Having autism does not mean your son cannot have a fulfilling life; do not allow the language of victimhood into your vocabulary. Use empowering words that teach him that he is without limits.

690. Work to give your child some structured chores he can work on each day. This will help increase the structure in his day and give him a feeling of accomplishment each day. We suggest placing play items in a home bin and helping with laundry.

691. Now these chores may not be easy to define or organize at first, but stick to it, let him have some responsibility and build on it. You may feel compelled to do the task yourself, but give him time to get the hang of it and you'll both be rewarded. As with any facet of this battle, you will need a little patience.

692. If you are completely honest with yourself about your child's strengths and weaknesses, you can more effectively advocate on his behalf. Self-delusion is a luxury you can't afford.

693. Get control of your children while they are still little. What's bearable when they are three isn't so bearable when they have pubic hair.

—Judith Chinitz, MS, MS, CNC, author of *We Band of Mothers*

694. A clearly defined daily schedule for your son can work wonders to remove uncertainty and accompanying frustration, for you both!

695. Don't get caught in the heat of the moment. When speaking, always take a breath and deliver a measured response.

696. If your selected task or chore is a compound one, break it up to achieve better compliance. Giving intermediate goalposts creates more opportunities for engagement and feelings of accomplishment.

697. Seek some good self time and solace. Go for a walk in the woods, run in the park, or read a book by a lake. You need to take care of yourself and activities in nature have a tonic effect.

698. Be flexible regarding timing. If your child moves away from brushing his hair, rather than forcing or pushing it, wait ten minutes and try again.

699. Flexibility is key, especially when it comes to timing. Knowing when to back off and when to return to a task or duty is more art than science. Keeping a flexible mindset and being persistent will help!

700. Try not to become overprotective. This is easy to do and easier to understand, but it is counterproductive. If you give your son control of a situation or at least expand his control of a situation, you can give him a "wow" moment where he can adapt and learn.

701. Keep yourself in a happy place. Easier said than done many times, I know. But your emotions have significant repercussions on your son, which should serve as a reminder and motive to keep things as positive as possible. Eliminate all negative influences, thoughts, and people if necessary. You and your son don't have time for negativity!

702. Communicate daily with your son's teacher or other school contacts to assess how behavior changes for the good or bad when in and out of school. He might be more regulated at school because of greater sensory opportunities via a swing or other OT equipment. You might be able to copy some, or remove other items that are helping or hindering.

703. Dealing with emotions is one of the more difficult areas for kids on the spectrum. One strategy you can follow is when your child gets emotional remember to "label" the emotion for him or her. Giving them a description of how they are feeling will help them to understand, learn and manage their feelings. This can be particularly useful in battling tantrums; just remember to work on the feelings after the child has calmed. You can use PECS or other visuals to describe the emotions if the child is non-verbal.

CHAPTER 62

Encourage Your Child to Succeed:
Building Self-Esteem

704. Raise your son to have good self-esteem, a necessary trait for a successful life. This means raising him with the firm knowledge that you love her and believe in him. Set high expectations for your boy, but give him the means to reach them. Teach him that he has the right to his own opinion, and respect the choices he makes when he is given the opportunity to choose. Raise him to believe that with hard work, he can reach his goals. In this way, he can reach his true potential.

—Chantal Sicile-Kira, www.chantalsicile-kira.com

705. Children develop most of their self-esteem based on what they hear and experience at home. Take a day and listen to the "messages" your boy is hearing at home. Does he hear mostly positive remarks or negative remarks? Is he accepted for who he is while still being expected to reach his potential? Is he complimented for all the positive things he does (and not just criticized for the negative behaviors)? Words and attitude do make a difference.

706. Parents should not allow autism to define their child. Just as one would not narrowly define a child with high blood sugar by saying "My child is diabetes," a child with autistic features and manifestations should not be labeled "autism." *Your child is not autism.* Your child is a sweet and wonderful individual who, just like all of us, has multiple positive attributes and a variety of challenges that need to be addressed.

—Dr. Mark Freilich, Total Kids Developmental
Pediatric Resources, New York City

707. Empowerment is the key to keeping children from becoming perpetual victims. If he can take care of himself, then adults should do nothing. If the child needs assistance, adults need to find whatever strengths or skills a child may have and build upon them.

—Ronald Mah, *Getting Beyond Bullying and
Exclusion PreK–5,* page 17

708. For their emotional and psychological health, you need to disappoint children: specifically to stress them; to allow frustration and failure; and to let them suffer while experiencing stress, frustration, and failure.

—Ronald Mah, *Getting Beyond Bullying and
Exclusion PreK–5,* page 17

709. Reframe academic and social challenges for children with AS so that challenged self-esteem can be regained through guided problem-solving.

—Ronald Mah, *Getting Beyond Bullying and Exclusion PreK–5,* page 17

710. Many children with autism are good at drawing, art, and computer programming. These talent areas should be encouraged. I think there needs to be much more emphasis on developing the child's talents. Talents can be turned into skills that can be used for future employment.

—Temple Grandin, PhD, author of *Thinking in Pictures* and *The Way I See It*; www.autism.com/ind_teaching_tips.asp

711. As much as possible, treat your children as though they were typically developing. Kids will always live up to your lowest expectations.

—Judith Chinitz, MS, MS, CNC, author of *We Band of Mothers*

712. Overly focusing on a child as if they are a problem to solve in order to be happy creates self-esteem issues. Resist this! Also, encouraging independence at each stage of development, even before the child seems ready, usually pays off in more success and stronger self-esteem.

—Lynette Louise, MS, Board certified in
Neurofeedback by BCIA, NTCB

713. Everyone is good at something. Ask your child to teach you something at which he or she excels while you may not. Does she have a natural golf swing? Make up her own songs? Role reversal that puts the child in charge is empowering.

—Ellen Notbohm and Veronica Zysk, *1001 Great Ideas
for Teaching and Raising Children with Autism Spectrum Disorders*

714. Go out in the community. Don't close your child in at home. Take your child to amusement parks, the zoo, or to visit friends and relatives.

715. Reward good behavior. Positive reinforcement can go a long way with autistic children, so make an effort to catch them doing something good. Praise them when they act appropriately or learn a new skill, being very specific about what behavior they're being praised for. Also, look for other ways to reward them for good behavior, such as giving them a sticker or letting them play with a favorite toy.

—Reprinted with permission from Helpguide.org. See www.helpguide.org/mental/autism_help.htm for additional resources and support.

716. Your kid will be limited by the aspirations you have. So, reach for the sky.

—Carole Harris, Joshua's Mom

CHAPTER 63

Making Sure Your Child Gets to Be a Kid

717. Downtime is key, for both you and your child. We lay out many options for therapies and activities in this book, but do remember to take a breather now and then. A little R and R from the battle is important.

718. Let your child be involved in picking an activity or two each week. Give him the responsibility of coming up with something that interests him and involves a trip away from the home.

719. Down and dirty. All kids need a chance to be carefree and playful. Let him run around and make a mess in the sandbox or dirt; deal with the mess later.

720. Make time for fun. A child coping with autism is still a kid. For both autistic children and their parents, there needs to be more to life than therapy. Find ways to play and have fun together. Don't obsess over whether or not these activities are therapeutic or educational. The important thing is to enjoy your child's company!

—Reprinted with permission from Helpguide.org. See www.helpguide.org/mental/autism_help.htm for additional resources and support.

CHAPTER 64

Responding to Undesirable Behavior

721. Just because your child has autism is no reason to steer clear of consequences for bad behavior. As with any child, he will smell weakness and take advantage if you let him get away with misbehavior.

722. Keep your behaviors in check. We are all prone to overreaction on occasion and these potentially intense outbursts (either positive or negative) can confuse and dysregulate your son. Keeping an even keel should be your focus.

723. Don't threaten a punishment you're not prepared to enforce. If you're not really going to cancel the birthday party, don't say you will. Don't count to three, or ten—your child will learn that he always has that long, and you didn't mean it the first time. If you teach a two-year-old, gently, but firmly, that you mean what you say, you don't have to keep teaching it—at sixteen, he will still know that you meant it the first time. Too often parents allow their children to push them around because they want to be liked, but your child will neither like nor respect you. Children crave boundaries.

724. Use positive discipline methods that work. Many parents use time-outs, yell, or take away privileges as their top three discipline options. If those methods aren't working for you, it can be frustrating, and can lead to more arguments if you're not feeling successful.
—Toni Schutta, M.A., L.P., Parent Coach, author, and founder of www.getparentinghelpnow.com

725.

Managing Severe Aggression
Tips by Cathy Purple Cherry, AIA, LEED AP

Our ASD son was physically aggressive from the age of 14 through now at the age of 19. His aggression was mostly displayed passively and through self-mutilation. On occasion, it was quite violent and sometimes directed towards his siblings. He has put his head and foot through a wall several times and punched himself to create blood and then bled all over the floor. Most recently, he attempted to stab himself with a big stick. My tips come from these past 5 years.

- The hardest lesson I had to teach myself was that an audience made the aggressive behavior of our ASD child worse. So, I learned to walk away, close the door, turn off the light, and ignore. It took me at least 3 years to get to this place.

- Prevention is possible in some cases especially when it comes to reducing conflict between the ASD child and their siblings. Violation of personal space is a major trigger. Thus, prevent path crossing and entering of each others' rooms. I would even orchestrate the best direction of travel around furniture to avoid conflicts.

- My son was famous for full body dropping as a negative and passive aggressive response. After he had self-mutilated, he would drop and shut down with no response whatsoever. If he was not in his own bedroom and, if I could, I removed him from our home and placed him on the grass in the yard. I watched from inside the house but absolutely did not let him know I was watching. Autistic children need time to learn to overcome their "fight" response.

- If your ASD child is violent, take him to the emergency ward at your hospital to have him temporarily committed to a psych hospital or call the police. Remove the threat from your home and inform others of what is happening.

- Medication changes can, at times, help. Do not hide these behaviors from your support team. Communicate immediately with your child's psychiatrist. Also, be aware that there is a calming medication that can be given just before these explosive episodes if you can see them coming. Again, speak with your child's psychiatrist.

CHAPTER 65

Working with Your Spouse

The following tips are adapted from an article by Toni Schutta, M.A., L.P., Parent Coach, author, and founder of www .getparentinghelpnow.com.

726. Reach an agreement to support each other publicly (or at least to remain neutral). You've heard about the importance of presenting a united front so your child can't divide and conquer, and it's true. It's confusing to your child when you argue about consequences in front of them. Children with a manipulative nature will use the situation to their advantage. Usually what happens is that you get embroiled in your own debate and the disciplinary action gets forgotten. It also undermines your spouse's parental authority in front of your child, which is something you don't want to do.

727. Develop a signal. Let's say that you strongly disagree with the other parent's choice of discipline. Agree ahead of time on a signal that you can give that means, "Take a break. Let's talk about this." Perhaps making a "T" sign with your hands to signal a time-out would be a good choice.

728. Talk privately about the child's offense and how it should be handled. There are few disciplinary actions that can't wait for a few minutes. Taking the time to leave the room and talk privately with your spouse about how to handle the situation is a respectful way of communicating to your spouse that there might be other options to consider. Regardless, you are setting a much-needed boundary that this is an adult matter, and that the two of you will handle it accordingly, as a team.

729. Check in with the other parent to see if they've already made a decision. Many children will use the one-liner, "Dad said that I could" to get what they want. When hearing this line from your child, a wise thing to do is to actually ask the other parent if she has already given approval to your child's request. Again, this demonstrates to your child that as parents, you are united and will support each other. Usually your child starts backpedaling if she is trying to manipulate you.

730. Develop three to four consistent family rules for the most-common misbehaviors. For instance, all families should have a rule that "No one's body will be hurt by hitting, kicking, biting, etc." Consistent discipline should be applied by both parents when physical aggression occurs. Parents will never agree on how to handle all offenses, but if parents respond consistently to the top three behaviors, it will make a significant impact.

731. Agree that smaller offenses can be handled at the discretion of the parent in charge. Once you have your family rules in place, try not to sweat the small stuff. It can be beneficial for children to learn different methods of problem-solving and communication, so if your spouse parents a little differently, it might actually benefit your child. For instance, some parents are better at using humor to move through tough situations, and if you're open to it, you can learn what works more effectively with each child.

732. Never say, "Wait till your father (or mother) gets home!" When a statement like this is made, it undermines the authority of the parent who says it, and makes the other parent the "bad cop." It's important that you both share equally in disciplining your children.

733. Don't blame the other adult. No one is to "blame" for the child's problems. Enlist the strengths of each member of the family, anyone who can help.

—Stanley I. Greenspan, MD, *The Supportive Family Environment*

CHAPTER 66

Defusing the Meltdown from Hell

734. When your boy is having a meltdown, try to remove others from the situation before trying to move the dysregulated child. It could help prevent the situation from escalating.

—Megan Miller, Head Teacher

735. Choices: Give your child a sense of control by providing choices that you are comfortable with.

—Jenn Gross, OTR/L

736. Practice deep breathing to help you stay calm during stressful times with your child. The calmer you are, the safer your child will feel, which can help prevent meltdowns from escalating even more.

—Jenn Gross, OTR/L

737. Set up a safe, small, quiet space that your child can use during times of frustration and anger. This gives them a comforting place of their own where they can retreat when they need a break.

—Jenn Gross, OTR/L

738. Ice: When battling the meltdown from hell, deploy ice! Chewing and holding ice can help calm your son down. He can also help in the creation and storage of ice in the freezer, giving him a reference point. Many boys will seek out a particular sensory input when on the verge of melting down; ice can serve as one more tool to help them self regulate. So remember, when in hell, freeze it over!

739. Anything added to systems already struggling to create and maintain stability can be overwhelming. "Anything" can mean perfumes, crowds (especially of children), household cleaning products, and even medications. Behavioral expectations beyond the person's ability are problematic.

—Carolyn Nuyens and Marlene Suliteanu, "The Holistic Approach to Neurodevelopment and Learning Efficiency (HANDLE)," *Cutting-Edge Therapies for Autism*

740. A "tantrum" or "meltdown" is actually a call for help, a plea to notice that the stress level has overflowed its container. A word of caution to family members: Try to identify what pushed your loved one beyond endurance—and don't expect it to always be the same thing. It could be noise in high-ceilinged supermarkets, or maybe it was the crowds, or smells, or any combination of these things. Always trust that there *is* a precipitating cause.

> —Carolyn Nuyens and Marlene Suliteanu, "The Holistic Approach to Neurodevelopment and Learning Efficiency (HANDLE)," *Cutting-Edge Therapies for Autism*

741. Parents who are dealing with their autistic child's problematic behaviors are encouraged to examine how they might be reinforcing them. For instance, the parents of an autistic child who tends to throw screaming tantrums throughout the day might be trying to put his tantrums on extinction. The parents might be successfully ignoring the tantrums while at home, but when he throws a tantrum at the playground, his parents might pick him up and bring him home to avoid creating a scene. Being picked up and carried home from the playground may in fact be reinforcing to the child, and therefore increase the likelihood that the tantrum behavior will continue.

> —Jenifer Clark, MA, PhD (c), "Applied Behavior Analysis," *Cutting-Edge Therapies for Autism*

742. Parents should work with schools in this regard, too; some children use this behavior as a way to get out of class or sent home, and if the school removes them, it just shows them they can get their way.

743. Parents must carefully evaluate their response patterns to be consistent with regard to problematic behavior.
—Jenifer Clark, MA, PhD (c), "Applied Behavior Analysis,"
Cutting-Edge Therapies for Autism

744. I have already mentioned the importance of keeping a journal or diary and provided a sample worksheet (www.skyhorsepublishing .com/Therapy_Logbook.xls) to do so. Here is another use for said log—analyzing the meltdown. If you note diet, time of year, day, weather, and such in this log and track meltdowns, you may uncover a pattern that can then be broken or at least prepared for. In my case I was able to determine that allergy season in the fall and spring alongside constipation would set Alex off. I am able to preempt many a meltdown with this knowledge.

745. Never try to teach during a meltdown. It won't work. Ask yourself how open you are to learning when you are angry, terrified, overwrought, overanxious, or otherwise emotionally disabled.

>—Ellen Notbohm and Veronica Zysk, *1001 Great Ideas for Teaching and Raising Children with Autism Spectrum Disorders*

746. When you sense a tantrum developing, shift gears and work to redirect your child's focus. Keep handy chewy toys, ice, or a favorite video, which may help nip a meltdown in the bud. Teach all your child's caregivers the warning signs and share strategies with them and other parents.

747. Ignore the tantrum. Seriously—this can work. Of course, it can only be applied at home. You could ignore a tantrum once you've brought him home from an off-site meltdown. A frustration meltdown has the best synergy with this strategy, as he will likely move on to something else, or just run out of steam. Then you can follow up with some queries as to what happened and try to understand what you can do to avoid this next time.

748. Again, keep an even keel. I know, easier said then done. But our kids are going to feed off our energy, good or bad, so work each day to keep it positive. Positive thinking may sound corny, but it does work and feeds upon itself.

749. During meltdowns, work to keep everybody safe. At home you can have some strategies in place. When out in the community this can become difficult and potentially drag others into it; it's best to remove your child from the location as quickly as possible.

750. Tantrums may scare you in their intensity, but they are typically a cry for help or understanding or even pain. It is a communication issue and your child is as afraid as you.

751. During the tantrum, offer support and comforting soothing words and actions. Do not however accede to demands made in the heat of the tantrum; it will only encourage further skirmishes.

752. Be wary of "simple" solutions. Don't accept a label for your child, or a single theory about a cause or cure.
　　　—Stanley I. Greenspan, MD, *The Supportive Family Environment*

Chapter 67

Adapting Your Career

753. If you do not have the option of taking a considerable amount of time off from work, [or if you are fully engaged with your career and would rather not interrupt it,] consider requesting an alternative work schedule. With an unconventional schedule, you could continue to do your work, but in a way that is conducive to your child's needs.

—Areva Martin, Esq., *The Everyday Advocate*

754. Work from home. If one spouse is able to transition to working from home, they could then be there for the child and provide flexibility for the family. Many folks telecommute nowadays.

755. Look into local jobs that provide flexible schedules so that you have easy access to your child at home or school, along with the schedule that allows you to accomplish what is necessary.

Section 9

....

Personal Care

E arly to bed and early to rise, makes a man healthy, wealthy, and wise.

—Benjamin Franklin as Poor Richard

CHAPTER 68

Toileting Skills

756. For children with autism, toilet training often occurs at only slightly later than expected ages for typically developing children ... For more moderately to severely impaired children, a good rule of thumb is to wait until non-language mental age is in the eighteen- to twenty-four-month age range.

—Bryna Siegel, *Helping Children with Autism Learn*

Toilet Training
Tips by Cathy Purple Cherry, AIA, LEED AP

757. Children with autism often learn through constantly repeated routines. Thus, the solution to successful toilet training may be tied to repeated practice. Be diligent. When you look back on the many years of rearing an ASD child to adulthood, you will realize "patience" was your child's gift to you! Thus ... practice and patience, practice and patience, practice and patience x hundreds of times.

758. An ASD child is not always aware of his surroundings. Their tactile sensitivities can be somewhat dulled. Our son is minimally affected by heat and cold, for example. Thus recognize that the child may not care if he has made a mess in his clothing. Acceptance by you of this behavior may be the bigger challenge and the only solution.

---

759. A reward system is known to be successful at school for modifying behaviors. Try a point sheet or rewards chart that leads to something good if your child takes steps towards successful toilet training. For our son, during a time in his development, a can of cherry pie filling was more motivating to him that an ice cream sundae so play to the interests at the time!

760. Develop a silent signal between you and your son so that he can quietly communicate his bathroom urges to you before accidents happen. If he uses this signal, reward him.

761. Try allowing your autistic child to pee in the grass. This can be fun for all little children and provides the ASD child the practice of not peeing in his pants.

762. If you are having problems with nighttime wettings, you may need to increase the frequency of bathroom visits. Set your alarm for every hour or two and bring him to the bathroom even if he appears to not have to go. As you get drier nights extend the time between visits until you are all good for the evening. Do not get discouraged by the occasional backslide. My son for years had this problem and in about a month I was able to transition him to no pull-ups and sleeping through the night.

763. FYI: Some meds, most notably risperidone/Risperdal, have the side effect of lessening urination control. Check your meds and review side effects.

764. When potty training a boy, the old "target in the toilet" often works, especially if a sibling or father joins in, and they see who can melt the ice cube first. Dad, be proud of your bathroom accomplishments; tell your wife how great you did, and let your son watch.

—Lynette Louise, MS, Board certified in
Neurofeedback by BCIA, NTCB

765. While ice works well, if you Google "toilet targets," or search on Amazon you will find several actual products that can be placed in the bowl to provide a visual target and potentially be fun for your son.

766. Some children who tend to remove all their clothing in the bathroom are simply taking extreme steps to prevent getting their clothes dirty. Careful work on toileting technique and rewards for good performance can help.

—*Autistic Spectrum Disorders: Understanding the Diagnosis & Getting Help* by Mitzi Waltz. Published by O'Reilly Media, Inc. Copyright © 2002 Mitzi Waltz. All rights reserved. Used with permission.
http://oreilly.com/medical/autism/news/tips_life.html

767. Some children might also want to have flushable wet wipes available to improve their after-toilet cleanup, and thereby avoid dirtying their clothes. Wipes can be purchased in small, discreet containers that fit well in a purse or backpack.

—*Autistic Spectrum Disorders: Understanding the Diagnosis & Getting Help* by Mitzi Waltz. Published by O'Reilly Media, Inc. Copyright © 2002 Mitzi Waltz. All rights reserved. Used with permission. http://oreilly.com/medical/autism/news/tips_life.html

768. While any child can have difficulty learning to be potty-trained, with autistic children, the process can be especially daunting. This doesn't mean that it is impossible, however. If you accept the challenges ahead of you, and maintain that you will overcome them to achieve positive results right from the very start, then you will ultimately be successful.

—Rachel Evans, ezinearticles.com/?Autism-and-Potty-Training-Tips---Getting-Through-this-Difficult-Time&id=643362

769. A common problem is that a child might be able to use the toilet correctly at home but refuse to use it at school. This might be due to a failure to recognize the toilet. Hilde De Clercq from Belgium discovered that an autistic child might use a small nonrelevant detail to recognize an object such as a toilet. It takes detective work to find that detail. In one case a boy would only use the toilet at home that had a black seat. His parents and teacher were able to get him to use the toilet at school by covering its white seat with black tape. The tape was then gradually removed and toilets with white seats became recognized as toilets.

—Temple Grandin, PhD, author of *Thinking in Pictures* and *The Way I See It*; www.autism.com/ind_teaching_tips.asp

770. If bedwetting remains an issue, rule out allergic bedwetting. If nighttime soiling is a problem, consult a knowledgeable gastroenterologist who has experience with children with autism. This might be a symptom of a gastrointestinal disorder.

CHAPTER 69

Bathing Skills

771. There are showering/bathing and bathroom routine PECS cards you can buy to hang in the shower and place on the bathroom wall. Use them to help your child build independence with his bathroom routines.

> —Kim Stagliano, Mom to three girls on the spectrum

772. Parents have a powerful weapon in their fight against autism: water. The bathtub, shower, or pool can offer countless opportunities to tame transitional stresses, promote social encounters, correct out-of-kilter motor systems, and promote sensory integration.

> —Andrea Salzman, "Aquatic Therapy,"
> *Cutting-Edge Therapies for Autism*

773. Parents who are greeted with unceasing crying jags every evening at bath time can try this trick for co-bathing. Take a towel, swaddle the child, offer the child the bottle, and then lower the child into a warm bath cradled in your arms. This works best if the child can be handed to an already-positioned parent ready in the tub. The transition is smoothed by the act of swaddling, immersion in skin-temperature water, and positioning in the cradling/nursing position. Yet, the child is successfully making a transition. Over time, the props can be removed and the transition can become more dramatic.

—Andrea Salzman, "Aquatic Therapy,"
Cutting-Edge Therapies for Autism

The following tips are adapted from *Autistic Spectrum Disorders: Understanding the Diagnosis & Getting Help by Mitzi Waltz*. Published by O'Reilly Media, Inc. Copyright © 2002 Mitzi Waltz. All rights reserved. Used with permission. http://oreilly.com/medical/autism/news/tips_life.html

774. This is a problem area with teenagers more often than it is with young children, according to parents. You might have to institute a schedule, or even allow gym-class showers to suffice during the school year.

775. Even for older kids, tub toys, soap "paints," bubble bath, or other items might allow you to get them in and out of a warm tub once a week.

---

776. Contrary to popular belief, it's not necessary to bathe children daily unless there are special medical or sanitary reasons to do so. Use a washcloth to zap any particularly grungy areas daily, and schedule an unavoidable bath time for one or more days each week. A flexible shower hose can be very useful for washing the hair of children who are afraid of the big shower.

777. Some kids who won't go near a bathtub will go swimming, which usually comes with the added bonus of a mandatory shower. In a pinch, you can see if they'll run through a lawn sprinkler in a pair of shorts. The novelty of pools and sprinklers sometimes trumps the fear of getting wet.

CHAPTER 70

Dental Hygiene at Home

778. Be persistent with toothbrushing, even if it is difficult. Be sure to make brushing teeth a routine part of your child's routine, morning and night. Start by counting to ten slowly while brushing so that your child knows when it will be over. Gradually add more time so that you are able to brush the entire mouth well.

—Ruby Gelman, DMD

779. Water is a great help to keep the mouth clean after meals. Drinking a few ounces of water after a meal can significantly reduce the acid buildup that begins with chewing and swallowing food. This can be a great help in preventing cavities.

—Ruby Gelman, DMD

780. Given our kids' sensory issues, you may have a tough time finding an acceptable toothbrush. Luckily nowadays there are many to try! Experiment with different bristles, head sizes, and those that vibrate. We have had success with the Oral-B battery-operated brushes; they make it a bit more fun and have the added benefit of being more effective.

781. When brushing your child's teeth, experiment with different brushing angles in order to be not only effective, but also comfortable enough from a sensory standpoint. Likewise, try different pastes and gels to get the right flavor and texture.

332

CHAPTER 71

Haircuts

782. If you can figure out what it is about haircuts that drives your child wild, then remove that particular trigger. You may then be able to get the job done at a regular barbershop or salon, with modifications. Common problems and solutions include:

783. Sensitivity to barbershop or salon odors: If this is the case, look for an old-fashioned barbershop that eschews smelly shampoos, or buy a home hair-cutting kit. Unscented products are often available, but you may have to buy them yourself and bring them in, or request them in advance.

784. Sensitivity to the sound of buzzing clippers or snapping scissors: Some people can tolerate one but not the other. There are also old-fashioned hand razors for cutting hair, but it's hard to find a barber who can wield one with precision. Call around! You might also try earplugs, or an iPod playing a favorite song through headphones. Your barber will happily work around headphones if it keeps the child in the chair. You might also choose to accept a longer hairstyle, if grooming is not a problem.

785. Sensory sensitivity in general. Try brushing the head and hair frequently with a medium-soft hairbrush. This may desensitize the area in time. You may be able to have your child sit in your lap during a haircut; a tight hug may calm him down. Again, home haircuts may be your best bet. Make sure you or your professional uses a neck strip and a cape to keep hair off the skin and clothes, and clean up with a soft brush and/or a blow dryer, set on cool. Parents whose children are of African descent may have a particularly hard time with sensory issues when it comes to hair care. Braided styles are the most convenient when it comes to grooming, but take a long time to achieve and involve a lot of pulling. Straightening chemicals and pressing are no picnic either. Short, natural styles may be the easiest to manage.

786. Extreme hyperactivity. One false move in the barber's chair can result in inadvertent punk-rock 'dos. Many parents swear by cutting hair while the child is fast asleep. Scissors work best for this operation. Keep a brush and comb handy, and work slowly. You may want to use a plastic bowl on the head to get an even length, or, for longer styles, hair tape (available at beauty-supply stores and many drugstores).

787. Some places will be flexible; it might help to go outside of usual business hours. Some that cater to children have DVD players. A massage during the cut can do wonders.

CHAPTER 72

Toenail and Fingernail Clipping/Cleaning

788. It may be an exaggerated fear of being cut, a desire to not lose a part of oneself, or the metallic clicking of the clippers, but many children with PDDs hate this grooming task. It's best if kids learn to do it for themselves as early as possible, although those with fine-motor problems may find it difficult.

—*Autistic Spectrum Disorders: Understanding the Diagnosis & Getting Help* by Mitzi Waltz. Published by O'Reilly Media, Inc. Copyright © 2002 Mitzi Waltz. All rights reserved. Used with permission.
http://oreilly.com/medical/autism/news/tips_life.html

789. Large, curved toenail clippers are easier to operate than small fingernail clippers and work fine for both fingernails and toenails. If possible, clip your child's nails while he is asleep.

790. Massage: You can get improved compliance with a bit of massage, and manage to work the clipping in.

Chapter 73

Personal Hygiene

791. Teach your child to count to ten when applying deodorant to ensure that enough product gets onto the underarms.

—Kim Stagliano, Mom to three girls on the spectrum

792.

- Most boys with autism do not learn what they need to know independently about hygiene and health, and this is an area that must be emphasized. Sometimes the lack of implementing has to do with the child having trouble remembering the steps or which routine to do when, and sometimes it is due to a lack of motor planning ability.

- If there are problems with self-care, it is important to do a task analysis of where your boy is having trouble (i.e., never washes his hair) and then figure out why (i.e., he's forgetful; has a sensitive scalp; hates the feel/smell of the shampoo; hard to lift his arms that high up). Once you know what the problem is, you can find a solution.

- Some boys like to wear the same thing over and over because of the feel of the fabric or the image on the shirt. This becomes unacceptable as they get older. Tell him these clothes can be worn at home, in private (i.e., not when special guests are over). Find some comfortable replacements that are appropriate for his age for him to wear out of the house.

- It's important to find a teen peer to go shopping with your son. You may think you know what is cool or "in," but a peer knows intuitively what the boys are wearing and what your son should wear. Looking like they fit in is really helpful, and encourages success in social situations with peers.

- Good hygiene needs to be addressed in boys early on, and good habits developed and emphasized. Explain why it's important (social stories tailored to ability level). There are health reasons (we need to do this to stay healthy) and there are social reasons (we need to stay clean in order to make friends).

CHAPTER 74

Clothing

793. Consider using 100 percent cotton clothing.

794. Wash clothing and bedding with nonallergenic soaps (no dyes, no additives).

The following tips are adapted from *Autistic Spectrum Disorders: Understanding the Diagnosis & Getting Help by Mitzi Waltz*. Published by O'Reilly Media, Inc. Copyright © 2002 Mitzi Waltz. All rights reserved. Used with permission. http://oreilly.com/medical/autism/news/tips_life.html

795. What do you do with a child who strips off his clothes at every opportunity? First, you try to find out why. The most common reason is sensory sensitivity, so first talk to an occupational therapist about instituting a program of sensory integration therapy.

796. In the meantime, see what you can do to make staying clothed more comfortable. Verbal children may be able to explain what they don't like about wearing clothes. Common problems include chafing waistbands, itchy fabrics, "new-clothes" smell, and annoying tags. Kids who can't stand regular waistbands can often handle elastic-waist pants and shorts, especially those made with soft fabrics, such as sweatpants. Others can wear only overalls or coveralls with ease, and these have the added "bonus" of being harder to remove.

797. For children who wear diapers, the diaper itself may be the problem. Check for and treat any actual diaper rash. (Incidentally, diaper rash can be caused by a yeast infection on the skin, which may indicate a larger problem with yeast overgrowth.) Experiment with different types of cloth diapers, various brands of disposables, and larger diapers if tightness around the waist and legs is an issue.

798. Over-the-diaper or training pants, sweatpants, overalls (especially the ones with snaps along the inseam), coveralls, and jumpsuits all work well. Some parents actually stitch down the overall straps each morning, or replace easy-open fasteners with something more complex. It's possible to open overalls and coveralls for larger children along the inseam and add unobtrusive snaps or Velcro for easy toileting without complete clothes removal.

799. Shirts that button up the back are also hard to remove.

800. Explore catalogs that carry special clothing for children with disabilities. Many items in these catalogs are especially good for older children who have toileting problems, or for children with orthopedic impairments in addition to an ASD.

801. Many people with sensory problems prefer soft fabrics, such as cotton jersey or terrycloth, over stiff fabrics like denim. If this is the case with your child, go shopping with that in mind. It can help to wash new clothing a few times before wearing it, to remove that stiff feeling as well as any unfamiliar smells.

802. Alternatively, some children complain that very soft fabrics feel "like dust."

803. If an aversion to clothing crops up suddenly, make sure you haven't just changed your detergent or fabric softener. There may be a smell or allergy issue going on.

804. Remove tags from inside of garments as needed.

805. One solution that will save you money and hassles is purchasing used clothing instead of new ones. These presoftened garments may already feel "just right." Again, they may need to be washed a few times to take away any bothersome scents.

CHAPTER 75

Puberty

806. In my case, the anxiety seized me for no good reason. Many people with autism find that the symptoms worsen at puberty. When my anxiety went away, it was replaced with bouts of colitis or terrible headaches. My nervous system was constantly under stress.

—Temple Grandin, PhD, *Thinking in Pictures*

807. Boys who do not like change may get upset when they see their body beginning to change and grow differently, and they realize they have no control over it. Explaining that everyone's body changes, and showing baby, children, teen, and current photos of adult family members will help them understand that puberty and growing happens to everyone.

808. Make sure to use correct names of body parts (i.e., penis, vagina), but also teach the synonyms that they may hear from others (i.e., boobs).

809. Explain that some changes will only be associated with the same sex (e.g., a boy will not begin to grow breasts, but a girl will), and this needs to be explained to both boys and girls. Explain that hair will only grow in certain places (the child may think the whole body eventually becomes progressively covered in hair, like a werewolf). Explain that extra hair just grows on the underarms and on the pubic area in women. Explain that on men, extra hair grows on the underarms and on the pubic area, and on the chest, face, and chin.

810. One out of four teens with autism is at risk of developing seizure activity during their adolescent years, possibly due to hormonal changes in the body. The seizures may be associated with convulsions, and others may be minor and not detected by simple observation.

811. When boys reach puberty and start showing more noncompliant behaviors, many parents think "Oh no—his autism is getting worse!" Actually, noncompliance is normal teenage behavior. At this point, parents need to remember to give the teen more choices in which to express himself and to have more control over some aspects of his day, within defined limits.

812. Precocious puberty has been estimated to be twenty times higher in children with neurodevelopmental disabilities, including autism.

813. It is important to begin teaching boys about their changing bodies *before* they hit puberty. Teaching them about the changes that will occur in the girl's body as well as their own body is important. Otherwise, they may be surprised by the changes they see in their female classmates, and not understand why they look different if they have not seen them for some time (i.e., summer vacation).

814. Puberty can be a difficult time for a boy on the spectrum, as usually they like predictability and routine, and many have a difficult time with change. Many have a hard time with the fact that their body is growing and changing and there is nothing they can do to stop it.

815. Drugs and alcohol: Alcoholic drinks or drugs often react adversely with your child's prescriptions, so you have to teach your teen boy about these dangers. If your son is very rule-oriented, try emphasizing that drugs and alcohol are illegal.

—www.yourlittleprofessor.com/teen2.html

816. Fathers, or other male "father figures," should be an integral part of teaching their boys about their bodies, hygiene, and sexual health. Don't assume that mothers know and can teach everything. These are topics where firsthand experience is crucial!

—Lauren Tobing-Puente, PhD, Licensed Psychologist,
www.drtobingpuente.com

817. When speaking to your child about his anatomy, be sure to use anatomically correct names for the parts of his body. Using incorrect terms could lead to confusion as he gets older.

—Megan Miller, Head Teacher

CHAPTER 76

Masturbation

818. Masturbation is normal teenage activity; however, most teenagers know to masturbate in private. Not so for boys on the spectrum. Parents need to teach their teenage boys the concept of private and public, and that masturbation is a private activity, not a public one.

819. If a teenage boy is attempting to masturbate at school, the best thing to do is redirect. At home, teens should be allowed a private place (their bedroom) to masturbate, and should be redirected there if they attempt to masturbate elsewhere in the house.

820. Touching in the genital area should be addressed as soon as it shows up regardless of age or gender. Just say matter-of-factly: "Touching your penis (or vulva) is for private time. Please wait till you are in bed at night." There is no room for emotions here. If you are vague or nervous, your child will likely continue to grow more inappropriate. Be clear and nonjudgmental. It works well.

—Lynette Louise, MS, Board certified in
Neurofeedback by BCIA, NTCB

Chapter 77

Sexuality and Sex Education

821. Don't be afraid to address sexuality and sexual behavior with children and adolescents who have autism, as they have the same basic human needs like everyone else. Failure to address this subject matter can lead to confusion, inappropriate behavior, and/ or things that can be both physically and emotionally damaging. Start educating children with autism about their sexuality early on. It is most beneficial when the information comes from their parent/caregiver.

—Dr. Mary Jo Lang

822. Reassure the child/adolescent that these feelings and desires are common, and it's okay to be experiencing them. Encourage them to ask questions and not to be embarrassed.

—Dr. Mary Jo Lang

823. Determine your comfort level in discussing sexuality and sex with your teenage son. Look for resources and specialists if you feel it would be helpful to you. Determine where your boy is at in his development. Obtain social and emotional age-appropriate materials to use while teaching him what he needs to know.

824. If the teenage boy is physically mature but delayed socially and emotionally, but is also gregarious, communicate openly and consistently with the boy's teachers, care providers, and, if appropriate, with local authorities, on where the boy is at in development, as well as what you are teaching them. This will help prevent social and/or legal issues arising from any possible inappropriate public behavior.

825. Teach your son early and often the basics about sexual awareness: What is sex, what is acceptable behavior, and when is it acceptable? Teach about boundaries: What boundaries should we have for our bodies, as well as when interacting with others?

826. Hypersensitivity or hyposensitivity due to sensory processing challenges may affect how a man with autism handles sexual intimacy. Extreme sensitivity may make it difficult for some young men to enjoy the physical aspects of a close relationship.

827. If your son sits in on sex education classes offered at the school for the mainstream population, he may hear all the facts but not personalize the information and realize that it is meant for him. This means that as a parent, you will need to verify that he has understood how this information relates to him.

828. Children and adolescents with autism tend to interpret things literally. Be clear and direct when discussing sexuality. Obtain materials that are socially and emotionally age-appropriate as well as anatomically correct when teaching your child/adolescent about sexuality and sexual behavior. Discuss the following topics with your child/adolescent: puberty, body parts, personal care, medical examination, social skills, and responsibilities surrounding sexual behavior.

—Dr. Mary Jo Lang

829. Address self-protection skills that encourage children and adolescents with autism to say "no" and to avoid individuals who seek to take advantage of them. It has been reported that children with disabilities are 2.2 times more likely to be sexually abused, making self-protection skills important to address and develop.

—Dr. Mary Jo Lang

Section 10

....

Safety

The best offense is a good defense!

CHAPTER 78
Personal Safety

830. Teaching the concept of "private" to little boys will help them understand important rules of private vs. public behavior. As they get older, it's important to have additional conversations about the topic, to help them understand rules of personal safety. At home, teach your son that it is okay to have clothes off in private areas of the house (i.e., their bedroom), but that in public areas of the house (living room, kitchen, etc.), they must keep their clothes on. Use picture icons if needed.

831. Relationship boundaries are difficult concepts for boys on the spectrum and must be taught and practiced. First, your boy needs to learn about different types of relationships (i.e., husband, wife, close friend, colleague, neighbor, shopkeeper). Then, he needs to be taught the concept of appropriate types of conversations and behaviors for the different relationships.

832. Boys on the spectrum need to know what constitutes sexual abuse. Nonverbal children and teens are at a high risk for sexual and physical abuse because of the perception that they are unable to communicate what happens to them. They are often grouped in classrooms or camp situations where predators know they can find victims.

833. Boys on the more able end of the spectrum are at high risk for sexual abuse because they are not good at figuring out people's intentions (i.e., picking up on nonverbal cues). This is why it's important for them to be taught what constitutes a sexual act and what is appropriate and inappropriate behavior.

834. It is important for the boy's safety that he be able to identify places on her body where it is inappropriate to be touched by others. It is important that the boy be able to communicate to someone when he has been touched in an "off-limits" area on his body. Off-limits areas of the body are those normally covered by a bathing suit.

835. Boys need to learn what sex is, and what constitutes a sex act. Boys with Asperger's and on the more able end of the spectrum are more apt to be victimized by others because of their gullibility. If they know what constitutes a sex act and they understand about when it is appropriate or not to engage in sexual acts, they are less likely to be victimized.

REPEAT TIP! Address self-protection skills that encourage children and adolescents with autism to say "no" and avoid individuals who seek to take advantage of them. It has been reported that children with disabilities are 2.2 times more likely to be sexually abused making self-protection skills important to address and develop.

—Dr. Mary Jo Lang

836. Never, ever tell a child on the autism spectrum to always obey grown-ups, especially if he has a hard time revising the rules as he gets older.

—Tara Marshall

Chapter 79
Home Safety

The following tips are adapted from *Autistic Spectrum Disorders: Understanding the Diagnosis & Getting Help by Mitzi Waltz*. Published by O'Reilly Media, Inc. Copyright © 2002 Mitzi Waltz. All rights reserved. Used with permission. http://oreilly.com/medical/autism/news/tips_life.html

Childproofing Dangerous Items

837. Most parents of crawling babies and toddlers take pains to remove hazards from their reach. You might need to continue and even expand this program with a child who has an ASD.

838. Funding may be available through government developmental-delay or mental health departments or private agencies to help cover the expense of these home modifications.

Items that can pose dangers include:

839. **Glass items and windows.** Some children seem to enjoy the sound of broken glass. This may necessitate using window treatments that can be locked down, or even boarding up some windows. Cutting a piece of foam to fit within the interior window well is an inexpensive solution that has worked for some parents. Replacing the glass in windows or picture frames with unbreakable plastic may prevent accidents.

840. **Window-blind cords.** These present a danger of hanging if the child puts his head inside the loop. Simply cut through the loop. For persistent offenders, you may want to cut the cords very short as well.

841. **Exposed electrical outlets.** A variety of plugs and covers are available for these.

842. **Exposed electrical wiring and extension cords.** Obviously, any exposed wires should be walled off somehow. Extension cords can either be eliminated by adding additional wall outlets or stapled to the wall. Rubber channels are available for making them inaccessible; these can usually be found at office supply stores.

843. **Electric fans.** Box fans are less dangerous, but little fingers may still fit in through the openings. Experiment with fan placement. You might consider using ceiling fans, swamp coolers, or air-conditioning instead in hot weather.

844. **Stove burners.** Burner covers can eliminate the attraction of fire or glowing coils, but can also cause burns if touched when hot. Some parents remove the knobs from their stove, place a barrier in front of the stove, add a disconnect valve for the gas behind the stove, or unplug it when not in use. Another option: Add locking doors to the kitchen.

845. **Lock up matches, lighters, and combustibles.** Watch out for guests who carelessly leave lighters or matches on tables.

846. **Household cleaning supplies, paints, solvents, and other chemicals.** A securely locked cabinet is a must if your child tastes and smells everything. Some young autistic children have incurred serious brain damage by repeatedly sniffing gasoline, glue, or other solvents. Of course, these items are sometimes abused as drugs by adolescents and teens.

847. **Medications, including herbal remedies and vitamins.** Most people are unaware that aspirin and Tylenol top the list of medication-overdose causes; in other words, keep everything that's medicine out of reach. Securely locked bathroom cabinets can work, but storing medications in the bathroom is actually not that great an idea due to the moisture level. You might install a similar cabinet in another room, or use a simple lock-box. Small cash boxes work well and are available at office supply stores for a reasonable price.

848. For the sake of convenience, you may wish to keep one week's worth of medications, supplements, and vitamins counted out in a plastic pill box, and then keep the pill box in your purse or another more-secure location. Be especially wary about leaving chewable medications and vitamins within reach.

849. **Houseplants.** A few are out-and-out poisonous, but heavy pots coupled with tantalizing fronds and tendrils can lead to injured heads and major messes. Use ceiling hooks to hang trailing plants well out of the way, or try using sticky-back Velcro or foam to secure pots to a flat surface.

850. **Cigarettes.** You would think they'd taste too horrible to eat, but some kids will do it. Tobacco can be quite dangerous when eaten. Keep cigarettes, cigars, chewing tobacco, and full ashtrays under wraps.

851. **Alcohol.** It's dangerous to mix even a little with many of the medications used for PDDs, and it has plenty of inherent dangers of its own. If you like to keep a selection of liquor, wine, or beer at home, you might consider a locked liquor cabinet, or keeping a separate refrigerator in a locked garage or basement.

852. **Cat litter boxes.** Cat feces carry disease and should not be handled by pregnant women or anyone with immune-system problems. The covered boxes may or may not be less attractive to marauding children. Protect the room where the cat box is with a baby gate, or add a cat door to a locked door.

853. **Stairs and stair banisters.** Baby gates or locked doors at the top and/or bottom of stairs may be enough. If the stairs need to be available to your child, make sure that any slats and banisters are too closely spaced for heads or bodies to slip through. If they aren't, you could add more slats or change the banister's style or position.

854. **Guns and other weapons.** These do not belong in the homes of children with neurological disorders, particularly teenagers. The combination of a high potential for depression and easy access to lethal force is very dangerous, and younger children with PDDs may be at risk simply due to their impulsivity. As some recent, tragic cases have shown, storing guns in a locked box under the parents' bed or in a gun cabinet does not guarantee safety around determined teens. If you enjoy shooting sports or hunting, see if you can store your guns at a shooting range or hunt club.

855. **Knives.** Sharp knives are common household tools, of course, but they also pose dangers. A drawer latch may be sufficient for keeping kitchen knives out of reach, or you may need to install a keyed lock on the knife drawer. Watch out for knives and other sharp kitchen tools that may be left in the sink, on countertops, or in the dishwasher.

856. Typical child locks for cabinets work for some children with autism. However, harder-to-open locks may be necessary for others. The Tot Lok system is the best thing for parents with smart, strong children. It is simple to open with the magnet lock, cannot be muscled open because it holds the door flush when closed, locks automatically when the cabinet closes, and can also be easily disabled if needed. Having spare keys hidden away is a good idea, and you can find some on eBay or at thrift stores.

—Candi Summers, Autism & Parenting Examiner, Examiner.com, http://exm.nr/9SfVh8

857. Stove safety is a big issue, and tiny plastic shields do not help when you have a child who is curious and taller than the stove. For those with children who simply will not leave it alone, you can go so far as to install the expensive but fully effective ($400) stove guard machine that disables the stove unless the right password is entered. Obviously this is not the solution for everyone, but if your child has a history of dangerously playing with the stove, it might be worth it. (www.examiner.com/ autism-parenting-in-dallas/heavy-duty-childproofing-tips-for-those-with-special-needs-children)

—Candi Summers, Autism & Parenting Examiner,
Examiner.com, http://exm.nr/9SfVh8

858. For the sneaky eater you can install a padlock on the fridge door or chain locks on cabinets. You can also put medicine and cleaning supplies inside a locked cabinet with a Tot Lok on it.

—Candi Summers, Autism & Parenting Examiner,
Examiner.com, http://exm.nr/9SfVh8

859. Plastic outlet covers might as well have a big sign on them that says PLAY WITH ME when a child with autism is involved. Not only are they useless at keeping fingers away from outlets, but sometimes, they actually encourage kids to play with the outlet because of the pleasant way they fit inside the plug. Outlet and switch covers that actually padlock can easily be installed, although they pose the typical dilemma of making it hard for parents to access them also.

—Candi Summers, Autism & Parenting Examiner, Examiner.com, http://exm.nr/9SfVh8

860. What about childproofing your SOFA? Children with sensory issues can be extremely rough on furniture, and with various potty accidents and a few "food exploration" incidents your sofa can take a beating and lose. IKEA has an excellent sofa and love seat series called Klippan. They are solid pieces of furniture that will take a beating and keep going. I recommend getting the slightly more expensive canvas cover, but the nylon covers have the appeal of being more water repellant. The slipcover that can easily be thrown in the washer is a major selling point. You can even replace the whole cover fabric if you grow tired of it. The final kicker is the price. With generously large sofas starting at $349, you can have a smart looking piece of furniture that you aren't so worried about replacing should an unmitigated disaster happen. The love seats fit three adults handily and can cost as little as $230. No removable cushions and a low back and sides that are fully cushioned add to the appeal of the Klippan as they lessen the likelihood of injuries to children who like to climb and take things apart.

—Candi Summers, Autism & Parenting Examiner,
Examiner.com, http://exm.nr/9SfVh8

Chapter 80

Runners

The following tips are adapted from *Autistic Spectrum Disorders: Understanding the Diagnosis & Getting Help by Mitzi Waltz*. Published by O'Reilly Media, Inc. Copyright © 2002 Mitzi Waltz. All rights reserved. Used with permission. http://oreilly.com/medical/autism/news/tips_life.html

861. If escapes are a problem for your family, please consider using the services of a professional security consultant. You may be able to get help from government developmental-delay or mental health agencies, or private agencies, to find and even pay for these services. Most people don't wish to turn their homes into fortresses, but in some cases, it's the most caring thing you can do. It could very well save a life.

862. Double- or triple-bolt security doors can slow down a would-be escapee, and some types can be unlocked only from the inside with a key. While expensive, they are tremendously jimmy-proof. Keep the keys well hidden, of course—on your person, if need be. Fire regulations may require that an exterior-lock key be secured in a fire-box or stored at the nearest fire station in case of emergency.

863. Bars can also be placed on windows, as many homeowners in urban areas already do. Like key locks, these can be a fire hazard. A security consultant, or perhaps your local fire department, may be able to come up with ideas. Some types of bars have interior latches.

864. Alarms are available that will warn you if a nocturnal roamer is approaching a door or window. Other types only sound when the door or window is actually opened. Depending on your child's speed, the latter may not give you enough response time.

865. Obviously, fences and gates are a good idea for backyards. Some types are less easily scaled than others. Although it might seem cruel, in extreme cases a child's safety could be secured by using electric fencing (usually this involves a single "live" wire at the top of a tall fence). Electric fencing kits are available at some hardware stores or at farm-supply stores.

866. For gates, key locks are more secure than latches.

867. Electronic locks of various types are another option, including remote-control and keypad varieties. These can be used for garage doors, gates, or exterior doors.

868. In some cities, the local police department is sensitive to the needs and special problems of the disabled. Officers may be available to provide information about keeping your child or adult patient safe and secure, whether he lives in your home, in an institution or group home, or independently in the community. Some also have special classes to teach self-defense skills to disabled adults.

869. A few police departments also keep a registry of disabled people whose behavior could be a hazard to their own safety, or whose behavior could be misinterpreted as threatening. Avail yourself of this service if your child is an escape artist, has behaviors that could look like drunkenness or drug use to an uninformed observer, uses threatening words or gestures when afraid, or is extremely trusting of strangers.

870. People with ASDs can have a bracelet or necklace made with their home phone number, an emergency medical contact number, or the phone number of a service that can inform the caller about their diagnosis. Labels you might want to have engraved on this item include:

- Nonverbal
- Speech-impaired
- Multiple medications
- Medications include . . . (list)
- Epilepsy (or other medical condition)

Members of the general public, and even some safety officials, may not know the word "autistic." They are even more unlikely to know what autistic spectrum disorder (ASD) or pervasive developmental disorder (PDD) means.

871. There are incredible programs out there like Project Lifesaver (www.ProjectLifesaver.org). Project Lifesaver has been commonly used with Alzheimer's patients, but has grown to address the needs of others, including those with autism, Down syndrome, traumatic brain injury, and more. People who qualify for the program are given a tracking device with a unique frequency to wear as a bracelet, which emergency responders can pick up and track with specialized equipment from one to several miles away. If your child has already gotten away from you—at home or in a public place—or you are afraid they will, see if there's a Project Lifesaver in your community and contact them. They do amazing work. There's almost always a wait list, so get on it if you qualify.

—Tim Tucker, "Practical Ideas for Protecting Autistic Children Before they Disappear," www.bothhandsandaflashlight.com /2010/04/16/practical-ideas-for-protecting-autistic- children-before-they-disappear

872. Look for a comfortable wrist or ankle band that will not irritate the child and is personalized with contact information and any emergency information (e.g. allergies, non-verbal). Should the band simply not work (for instance, if he will just not keep it on) you can purchase iron on labels to work into his clothing.

873. Know the signs. Your best defense against something terrible happening is to notice patterns in your child's behavior that might indicate they are about to try to escape or otherwise take off in a way that could put them in serious danger, such as running off a sidewalk into a street. Noticing any strong interests, especially ones that get more intense, might help in knowing when and where they might wander off to fulfill those interests.

—Tim Tucker, "Practical Ideas for Protecting Autistic Children Before they Disappear," www.bothhandsandaflashlight.com /2010/04/16/practical-ideas-for-protecting-autistic-children-before-they-disappear

Bonus Safety Tips

- Take the time to inform your local law enforcement agency and emergency personnel that a child with special needs resides at your home and may require special attention during an emergency.
- As with the tip above, inform your neighbors about your special needs child, especially if they are a runner. Providing photos and contact information can be a lifesaver.
- Visual symbols of Stop signs or other such signage can be used in the home and are easily purchased on the internet. Google "street signs" and you'll find plenty of options. These symbols can stall a child from taking flight.
- Using an alarm system, dead-bolts, and window locks are necessary to secure your residence, especially if your kid is a runner.
- As with infants, a speaker system or even a video monitor can serve to provide a level of comfort and help you transition a child into his/her own room.
- Fences and gates with tricky locks or combinations can help you secure your yard if your kid is a runner.
- A PDF, smart phone, or other device can serve to aid as in tracking down a runner. Learn to use the GPS function!

874. If you have a runner, know where in your neighborhood your child gravitates to. These will be the likely destinations. You can also increase your frequency of visits to these locations to lessen the fascination with them.

875. Swimming is not only great exercise for your child but can serve as a safety tool as well. Frequently, kids with autism favor water and water based activities. Keep your kid safe with some lessons!

876. Internal alarms: Everything depends on preventing your child from getting out in the first place. You want to build up multiple layers of "defense" against escape. If you can't stop your child from getting out of your house, slowing them down might buy you the time you need. If your child gets up and wanders around at night, install things that will either keep them in a defined area or that will notify you if they get outside that area. We have gates up around the house that are mounted directly to the wall; even most adults who visit us can't figure out how to open them. They could be hurdled by larger kids, of course. Some parents switch their child's bedroom doorknob around so it can be locked from outside the child's room. This does present a potential fire-escape hazard, though, so really think that through.

—Tim Tucker, "Practical Ideas for Protecting Autistic Children Before they Disappear," www.bothhandsandaflashlight.com /2010/04/16/practical-ideas-for-protecting-autistic- children-before-they-disappear

877. Door chimes / motion detectors. Most parents of children with autism worry about their child simply unlocking the front door and walking away. When your child is nonverbal this is especially worrisome, because if someone tries to help your "lost" child come home, they cannot tell the person their name or address. This issue can be dealt with in a multifaceted way, starting with a door chime. It offers the security of letting you know when the door has been opened. There are also motion-sensor chimes that let you know a person is in a specific area of the house, like the kitchen or the bathroom, helping avoid an incident altogether rather than installing useless locks on toilets and appliances that your child will bypass anyway. These items are surprisingly inexpensive, usually running around $25 each.

—Candi Summers, Autism & Parenting Examiner,
Examiner.com, http://exm.nr/9SfVh8

878. You can also get a permanent ink stamp for your child's clothing. You can skip trying to put tags or bracelets on children with sensory issues, but a laundry stamp on the inside (or even outside if it is necessary) doesn't feel like anything other than their regular clothing. Many laundry stamps that are self-inking only offer one line of type, but if you get laundry stamping ink, you can use it with any stamp, even one that has your full name, address, and phone number on it.

—Candi Summers, Autism & Parenting Examiner, Examiner.com, http://exm.nr/9SfVh8

879. If it's practical and financially an option, fence in your yard. This is a big expense, but consider it if possible. Giving our kids room to roam and play safely is important, too.

—Tim Tucker, "Practical Ideas for Protecting Autistic Children Before they Disappear," www.bothhandsandaflashlight.com /2010/04/16/practical-ideas-for-protecting-autistic-children-before-they-disappear

880. Set up "outdoor traps" in your yard or outside your apartment. I wish I could take credit for this idea, as it's brilliant. Here's where you can leverage your child's intense interests to great advantage. This particular parent's child loves pinwheels, so she put pinwheels on various objects and in the ground in strategic places in her yard. One time he got out, but he saw one of the pinwheels and just stood there playing with it rather than continuing to run. It bought her the minute or two she needed to find him and stop him from going any farther. Figure out how to take your child's interests and convert them into a system that will at least stall them or keep them from going any farther.

—Tim Tucker, "Practical Ideas for Protecting Autistic Children Before they Disappear," www.bothhandsandaflashlight.com /2010/04/16/practical-ideas-for-protecting-autistic-children-before-they-disappear

881. Determine where in your neighborhood your child might go first if they leave your immediate premises. Pay attention to what your child is most interested in around your neighborhood. Is it a particular neighbor's yard decorations? Is it a pool? Is it a playground? Is it someone's flowers? Is it a street sign? Think about what correlates to their interests, but also just note their expression as you go around the neighborhood. Do they perk up or stare a long time or appear very drawn to something in particular when you pass it? If so, write that down and commit it to a map. These landmarks will form your emergency search map of where to look first.

—Tim Tucker, "Practical Ideas for Protecting Autistic Children Before they Disappear," www.bothhandsandaflashlight.com /2010/04/16/practical-ideas-for-protecting-autistic-children-before-they-disappear

CHAPTER 81

Car Safety

882. Especially for younger kids, escaping from their car seat can be one of the worst problems we encounter. For kids still in the five-point harness, you can simply take the lap part that everything buckles into and flip it over such that the button is facing down into the child's lap. Everything still buckles together correctly in the models I've seen. That in itself might be enough. For other kids, especially those using the regular seat belt, there are covers available that make it difficult for them to get to that release button.

—Tim Tucker, "Practical Ideas for Protecting Autistic Children Before they Disappear," www.bothhandsandaflashlight.com /2010/04/16/practical-ideas-for-protecting-autistic-children-before-they-disappear

883. *Always* enable the child locks on the rear doors of your vehicle. If adult passengers riding in your backseat complain, tell them they can walk home.

—Tim Tucker, "Practical Ideas for Protecting Autistic Children Before they Disappear," www.bothhandsandaflashlight.com /2010/04/16/practical-ideas-for-protecting-autistic-children-before-they-disappear

884. Your local Autism Society has stickers available to members that you can put on your car window. This lets emergency responders know that your child is autistic and might not respond to any verbal instructions.

—Tim Tucker, "Practical Ideas for Protecting Autistic Children Before they Disappear," www.bothhandsandaflashlight.com /2010/04/16/practical-ideas-for-protecting-autistic-children-before-they-disappear

CHAPTER 82

Eliminating Household Toxins

The following tips are adapted from the article "Emerging Science Combined with Common Sense Gives Parents Better Options for Preventing Autism" by Maureen McDonnell, RN, *The Autism File*, Issue 35, 2010.

885. Switch to green cleaning and personal-care products (e.g., shampoo, toothpaste, body lotion, facial cream). The average American home contains three to ten gallons of hazardous materials, and 85 percent of the chemicals that are registered have never been tested for their impact on the human body. See the *Green This!* series of books by Deirdre Imus.

886. Eat organically grown grains, vegetables, fruits, nuts, meat, chicken, and eggs.

887. If a woman has taken many drugs—prescription or over-the-counter—or works or lives in a chemically laden environment, she might consider a detoxification or cleansing program.

888. Find a "green" dry cleaner (the chemical used in most dry-cleaning facilities, perchlorethylene, is a known carcinogen).

889. Use a stainless-steel water bottle to carry and consume filtered water. Heated or not, the soft plastic bottles will release phthalates. Antimony can also be released from polyethylene terephthalate.

890. For more information about water filters, call 1–800–673–8010 or visit NSF International's website, at www.nsf.org/Certified/DWTU/ and the Natural Resources Defense Council website at www.nrdc.org/water/drinking/gfilters.asp.

891. Safely remove mercury-based amalgam fillings with a dentist associated with the American Holistic Dental Association (www.holisticdental.org) at least six months before becoming pregnant, and not while breastfeeding.

892. Prior to conceiving, consult a natural health–care clinician or physician well versed in treating GI disturbances, as well as elevated levels of toxins and heavy metals. One option is to contact a naturopathic physician (ND) or an MD associated with the American College for Advancement in Medicine (www.acamnet.org).

893. Minimize consumption of large fish (for mercury levels of fish, check www.gotmercury.org).

894. To build beneficial microflora, take high-quality probiotics (in addition to improving levels of beneficial intestinal flora, these have been shown to decrease intestinal absorption of certain chemicals by facilitating their excretion) and consume more fermented foods. See www.BodyEcologyDiet.com.

895. Improve indoor air quality by opening the windows and creating cross ventilation.

896. When painting, choose low- or no-VOC (volatile organic compounds) paints. Select green building or remodeling products and allow adequate time for "non-green" building materials to outgas before moving back into the newly built or renovated nursery, room, or home. Reduce exposure to electromagnetic radiation by eliminating the use of microwave ovens, keeping cell-phone usage to a minimum, and storing your cell phone in your bag rather than in your pocket.

897. Do not sleep near a computer or other wireless device.

898. Use natural methods for controlling household and garden pests.

899. Have children avoid playing on pressure-treated wood decks and swing sets (source of arsenic).

900. Minimize the use of fire-retardant sleepwear (contains the toxic material antimony).

901. Purchase organic mattresses and linens.

902. Remove shoes before entering the home to prevent contaminants from soil coming into the house.

903. We think that many of the symptoms of autism may be related to problems caused by environmental toxins. We know autism has some sort of environmental component, and toxins can be neurologically damaging, so this is logical. Trying to correct the underlying metabolic abnormalities and using methods to remove environmental toxins can help our autistic children get better.

—Bryan Jepson, MD, Medical Director,
Thoughtful House Center for Children

904. Choose foods that are less processed and clean of chemicals and toxins. Why? Because children with autism are already compromised nutritionally. Use organic options whenever possible.

905. Tap water should be avoided, as it contains many different kinds of contaminants; invest in a good filtration system.

906. Avoid large fish, which have the highest concentrations of mercury; focus on freshwater species.

907. Avoid vaccines containing thimerosal.

908. Check your home for toxins such as lead and mold.

909. If you have a fireplace, avoid burning treated wood.

910. Tylenol hinders glutathione production. This is a good opportunity to mention that you should not give Tylenol to ASD kids at any time; it reduces glutathione, which they are usually deficient in, and which is needed in order for your immune system to work properly.

911.

There is substantial evidence to suggest that many children with autism suffer from exposure to mercury, and probably other toxic metals and toxic chemicals. The data includes:

- A literature review by Bernard S. et al. showed that the symptoms of autism were very similar to those of people suffering from infantile exposure to mercury poisoning.

- A study by James et al. found that children with autism had low levels of glutathione, which is the body's primary defense against mercury.

- A large study by Nataf et al. found that over half of children with autism had abnormal levels of a porphyrin in their urine that highly correlates with a high body burden of mercury.

- Two studies of airborne mercury, in Texas and in the San Francisco Bay Area, found that the amount of mercury in the air correlated with the incidence of autism.

- There have been nine epidemiological studies of the link between thimerosal in vaccines and autism. Four published studies by the Geiers have consistently found that children who received thimerosal in their vaccines had a two to six times higher chance of developing autism than those who received thimerosal-free vaccines. Four published studies by groups affiliated with vaccine manufacturers have failed to find a link, and one was inconclusive. Three of the studies were conducted in other countries where the usage of thimerosal is much less and the incidence of autism is much lower, so those results have limited relevance to the U.S.

—Dr. James B. Adams, "Chelation: Removal of Toxic Metals,"
Cutting-Edge Therapies for Autism

SECTION 11

....

Venturing Out

Upon venturing out you will undoubtedly run into ignorance. Here is a brief rejoinder I have found useful in New York City.

Your son is causing a bit of a ruckus while being out and about. A person, ignorant about autism, comments on your parenting skills and disobedient child. You walk away. Not bad, but every now and then, a rejoinder is necessary, for you (schadenfreude) and them (education), and your son (Mom/Dad has my back!). A proven quick comeback for these times: "Sorry, he is autistic. What's your excuse?"

CHAPTER 83

Dining Out

912. Avoid long—or, let's face it, any—restaurant waits. Go early or late to avoid any crowds. The last thing you want is a pre-meal meltdown! Try diners; we have found them to be accommodating, and they have a wide range of options.

913. Anyplace that has an outside seating option is great; less hassle with cleanup, should your son be a messy eater like Alex, and you can always take a walk.

914. Make sure the restaurant can accommodate whatever diet your child is on. This is not always easy. Google the menu and then call to confirm ingredients and how the meal you'll be ordering is prepared. Mention allergies, and make clear that MSG is off limits.

915. Once you find a good place that's suitable for your child, become a regular and tip well. In the future you'll be able to call and make special requests, or even order in advance!

916. You can ease your way into eating out. First, I took Alex to some out-of-the-way places just to get french fries. Then, I took him to restaurants at less-popular times and ordered full meals. Finally, we worked toward having a regular meal out at dinnertime. This takes time. To get him to a comfortable place dining out, I worked on this routine for about four months, leading up to his birthday. On the big day he was able to remain regulated, and I was able to actually enjoy eating out. Practice makes perfect.

917. You can also prepare for eating out by watching Elmo or other favorite characters eat out on TV or YouTube, and discussing how you will both be doing the same.

918. Once you are seated and you've ordered, pay your bill ahead of time. Give the waiter your card and mention the possibility of having to leave early.

919. As with travel, bring some items to help with any waits. YouTube on an iPhone works for us, but books and chewy toys can also serve the purpose.

920. Feel free to mention autism at the start of the meal to anyone working your table; it will help the staff understand, and you'll be able to relax.

CHAPTER 84

Vacations and Travel

921. Remember to plan your vacations around your child's interests. Alex loves the water and being outdoors, so I focus on places with a pool and access to hiking trails. You can usually plan many nice day trips to national parks or scenic local areas.

922. Vacation in a national park. Think about it: You bring your own food, so no worry about diet violations; it's cost-effective, beautiful, and a wonderful way to connect with your son and to nature. There is something soothing and stabilizing about hiking in the great outdoors. There are many fabulous parks located throughout the U.S. Check out www.nps.gov/findapark/index. htm.

"In every walk with nature one receives far more than he seeks."
—John Muir

923. Looking for a fun, family-friendly vacation? The Disney Corporation is very accommodating with special-needs children and their families. Head to the nearest Guest Services at any of the parks with a letter from a doctor, therapist, or teacher stating your children's special needs and challenges, and they will do their best to accommodate you with passes (so you don't have to wait in line), and if you're lucky, even a cast member to guide you!

—Julie Fishelson Mahan, MSW, LSW,

Note: Other theme parks, including SeaWorld and Busch Gardens, also have similar programs.

924. Some cruise lines now have cruises specially designated for children with autism and their families.

925. Plenty of rest time at the hotel is one of the keys to a successful vacation. And putting a cap on the number of activities per day should help to prevent meltdowns.

926. Ask your OT for an "on-the-go" sensory box to help your child proactively remain regulated on flights or long car trips. A shoe box or Ziploc with theraputty, Play-do, squish balls, etc., definitely comes in handy.

—Julie Fishelson Mahan, MSW, LSW,

927. Off-peak weeks at theme parks meaning shorter lines, smaller crows, and less noise. Plan accordingly. And don't forget to bring earplugs or headphones for your kid for when the loud noises get to be too much for him.

928. Asking a doctor, therapist, or teacher for a letter addressed to the airline that states the child's diagnosis and challenges can cut down on wait time getting on and off a flight. Being able to hand a typed letter to someone rather than talking about your child in front of them is always a better option, especially during difficult times in the air.

—Julie Fishelson Mahan, MSW, LSW,

929. Transitions are usually difficult for many on the spectrum, and traveling is really a series of transitions. Preparing the person—child, teenager, or adult—as much as possible will make any trip a more enjoyable experience for all involved. Some advance planning of specific steps of the trip can be made ahead of time to prepare both the person and the environment for a better travel experience.

—Chantal Sicile-Kira, www.chantalsicile-kira.com

Leaving the security of home for a new place can be off-putting for individuals with autism. How you prepare the person on the spectrum depends on his or her age and ability level. Here are some tips from Chantal Sicile-Kira (www.chantalsicile-kira.com):

930. Think of the individual's daily routine and the items he likes or needs and bring them along to make him feel more at home. Bring whatever foods and drinks will keep him happy on the trip, especially if there are dietary restrictions.

931. Buy some small, inexpensive toys or books that he can play with during the journey (and if you lose them, it won't be the end of the world). If he only plays with one favorite item, try to find a duplicate and see if you can "break it in" before the trip.

932. Do not wash any items (including plush toys) before the trip, as the individual may feel comfort in the "home" smell of his cherished item.

933. Put up a monthly calendar with the departure date clearly marked, and have the person check off every day until departure. Bring the calendar with you and mark off the number of days in one place or on the trip, always having the return date indicated.

934. Put together a picture and word "travel book" of what means of transport you are going to be using, who you are going to see, where you will sleep, and what you will do or see at your destination(s). Go over this with the person, like you would a storybook, as often as you like in preparation for the trip. Using a three-ring binder is best, as you can add extra pages or insert the calendar mentioned above for use on the trip.

935. Put together a picture or word schedule of the actual journey to take with you on your trip. Add extra pages to the travel book. Add Velcro and attach pictures or words in order of the travel sequence. For example, a picture to represent the car ride to the airport, going through security, getting on the airplane, etc. For car trips, pictures representing different stops on the trip and number of miles to be driven can be used. Add an empty envelope to add the "done" pictures when you have finished one step of the journey.

936. Taking a short trip before attempting longer ones is recommended, if possible. This will help the person get used to traveling and give you the opportunity to plan ahead for possible areas of difficulty. Also, if you use the travel book system, it will help the person make a connection between the travel book and any impending travel in the future.

Some preparations can be made ahead of time for the different environments and means of transport you will be using. Most people and companies in the field of tourism are willing to help to ensure a positive environment for all of their customers and guests. Here are some tips from Chantal Sicile-Kira (www.chantalsicile-kira.com):

937. When staying in a hotel, it is a good idea to call ahead and ask for a quiet room. You may wish to explain about the person's behavior if there is a likelihood of him or her exhibiting such behavior in the public part of the hotel. Same with a friend or relative's home; it can be a bit disconcerting for everyone concerned if your child or adolescent takes his clothes off and races through your friend's home stark naked.

938. If you are traveling by plane, call the airline as far in advance as you can, and tell them you will be traveling with someone who has special needs. Some airlines have "special assistance coordinators." You may wish to explain about the person's needs and some of the behaviors that may affect other travelers, such as rocking in their seat. If the person is a rocker, asking for bulkhead seats or the last row of seats on the plane will limit the number of fellow travelers that are impacted by the rocking. If you need assistance getting the person and luggage to the gate, or to change planes during the trip, call ahead and reserve wheelchair assistance. Even if the person does not need a wheelchair, this guarantees that someone will be waiting for you and available to assist you. (This was suggested to me by a special assistance coordinator when I told her that the help I had requested had not been provided on a recent trip). When requesting the wheelchair, you may need to explain about the person's autism. For example, I have explained in the past that my son with autism had difficulty moving forward in a purposeful manner and we needed help to get to the gate to catch a connecting flight.

939. Persons with autism should always carry identification. Make sure he has an ID tag attached to him somewhere, with a current phone number written on it. You can order medical bracelets, necklaces, and tags to attach to shoelaces. Additionally, if the person can carry it in his pocket, make an ID card with a current photo, date, and phone numbers. Be sure to include any other important information, such as allergies and medications, and any special information (i.e. nonverbal).

940. Adult passengers (eighteen and over) are required to show a U.S. federal or state-issued photo ID that contains the following information: name, date of birth, gender, expiration date, and a tamper-resistant feature in order to be allowed to go through the checkpoint and onto their flight. Acceptable identification includes: driver's license or other state photo identity card issued by the Department of Motor Vehicles (or equivalent) that meets REAL ID benchmarks (at time of writing, all states are currently in compliance).

·······························

Holidays, Birthdays, Gifts

You say it's your birthday. Well, it's my birthday too, yeah!

CHAPTER 85

Tips for Surviving the Holiday Season

The following tips are adapted from "Twelve Tips for Helping People with Autism and Their Families Have a Happy Holiday" by the Autism Society of America, www.autism-society.org/holiday_tips.

941. Preparation is crucial for many individuals. At the same time, it is important to determine how much preparation a specific person may need. For example, if your son has a tendency to become anxious when anticipating an event that is to occur in the future, you may want to adjust how many days in advance you prepare him. Preparation can occur in various ways, by using a calendar and marking the dates of various holiday events, or by creating a social story that highlights what will happen at a given event.

942. Decorations around the house may be disruptive for some. It may be helpful to revisit pictures from previous holidays that show decorations in the house. If such a photo book does not exist, use this holiday season to create one. For some it may also be helpful to take them shopping with you for holiday decorations so that they are engaged in the process, or involve them in the process of decorating the house. And once holiday decorations have been put up, you may need to create rules about those that can and cannot be touched. Be direct, specific and consistent.

943. If a person with autism has difficulty with change, you may want to gradually decorate the house. For example, on the first day, put up the Christmas tree; then on the next day, decorate the tree; and so on. And again, engage them as much as possible in this process. It may be helpful to develop a visual schedule or calendar that shows what will be done on each day.

944. If a person with autism begins to obsess about a particular gift or item they want, it may be helpful to be specific and direct about the number of times they can mention the gift. One suggestion is to give them five chips. They are allowed to exchange one chip for five minutes of talking about the desired gift. Also, if you have no intention of purchasing a specific item, it serves no purpose to tell them that maybe they will get the gift. This will only lead to problems in the future. Always choose to be direct and specific about your intentions.

945. Teach them how to leave a situation and/or how to access support when an event becomes overwhelming. For example, if you are having visitors, have a space set aside for the child as his safe/calm space. The individual should be taught ahead of time that they should go to their space when feeling overwhelmed. This self-management tool will serve the individual into adulthood. For those who are not at that level of self-management, develop a signal or cue for them to show when they are getting anxious, and prompt them to use the space. For individuals with more significant challenges, practice using this space in a calm manner at various times prior to your guests' arrival. Take them into the room and engage them in calming activities (e.g., play soft music, rub his back, turn down the lights, etc.). Then when you notice the individual becoming anxious, calmly remove him from the anxiety-provoking setting immediately and take him into the calming environment.

946. If you are traveling for the holidays, make sure you have your son's favorite foods or items available. Having familiar items readily available can help to calm stressful situations. Also, prepare him via social stories or other communication systems for any unexpected delays in travel. If you are flying for the first time, it may be helpful to bring him to the airport in advance and help him to become accustomed to airports and planes. Use social stories and pictures to rehearse what will happen when boarding and flying.

947. Prepare a photo album of the relatives and other guests who will be visiting during the holidays in advance. Allow the person with autism access to these photos at all times and also go through the photo album with him while talking briefly about each family member.

948. Practice opening gifts, taking turns and waiting for others, and giving gifts. Role-play scenarios with your child in preparation for him getting a gift he does not want. Talk through this process to avoid embarrassing moments with family members. You might also choose to practice certain religious rituals. Work with a speech-language pathologist to construct pages of vocabulary or topic boards that relate to the holidays and family traditions.

949. Prepare family members for strategies to use to minimize anxiety or behavioral incidents, and to enhance participation. Help them to understand if the person with autism needs calm discussions, and if he prefers to be hugged/kissed or not. Provide other suggestions that will facilitate a smoother holiday season.

950. If the person with autism is on special diet, make sure there is food available that he can eat. And even if he is not on a special diet, be cautious of the amount of sugar consumed. And try to maintain a sleep and meal routine.

951. Above all, know your loved one with autism. Know how much noise and other sensory input he can take. Know his level of anxiety and the amount of preparation it may take. Know his fears and those things that will make the season more enjoyable for him. Don't stress. Plan in advance. And most of all, have a wonderful holiday season!

Chantal Sicile-Kira (www.chantalsicile-kira.com) provides the following tips for surviving the holidays:

952. The winter holidays and celebrations can be difficult for children on the spectrum and their families. Some areas of difficulty include:

- The stores are full of noise, lights, lots of people, and winter holiday music that can create major overwhelm for those with sensory processing challenges.
- Social requirements such as visiting relatives wanting a hug or a kiss that can feel painful.
- Holiday dinners where he is expected to try foods or sit for long periods of time with so many people and so much commotion.
- Many children are mesmerized by the colors and textures of the ribbon and wrapping paper and do not open the present but stim on (get engrossed in playing with) the wrapping.
- The child does not understand personal space or have notions of safety and so he may run around the house or handle something breakable.
- Relatives may think the that the child is misbehaving, and may try to discipline the child, not realizing that the child really can't help it, and that discipline is not helpful when it comes to sensory overload and high anxiety.
- Parents have a difficult time because they know there are certain expectations of behavior that relatives and friends have and that the child cannot fulfill.

953.

What can you do? Here are some tips on how to prepare your friends and relatives whom you will be visiting:

- Explain the difficulties your child has with the holiday dinner environment, decorations, noise etc.
- Let your friends and relatives know that he is not just misbehaving, and that he is learning little by little how to handle these situations.
- Explain about dietary challenges so they don't expect him/ her to eat what everyone else is eating.
- Ask if there is a quiet room (child-proof in terms of décor) where your child can retreat for some quiet time to escape the commotion and noise.
- Send them a short but sweet letter or email explaining why your child acts the way he does and the difficulties of the holidays from his point of view. They will have a better understanding of why he won't wear a necktie, and why as more and more people start arriving, he tries to escape the room.

954. To prepare your child ahead of time:
- Make a social stories book about what will be happening and the behavioral expectations. If possible include photos of who he will be seeing and the house as it was decorated at last year's holiday season. If he is going to church, do the same for that environment.
- Play some of the music he may be hearing at this holiday season.
- Practice unwrapping presents—wrap a bunch of boxes up with his favorite treats inside and have him open them to get to them.
- Practice a handshake if he can tolerate that.
- Write rules together—i.e., how long he thinks he can tolerate sitting at table, and expected behavior.

955. On the day of the holiday celebration:
- Remind your child of the agreed upon rules.
- Pack some little toys he can play with in his lap at the dinner table.
- Bring some foods he can eat, especially if he is on a specific diet.
- Arrive early so that the noise level builds up slowly for him.
- Do not let the expectations of others ruin your day. Do what you need to do to make it as comfortable as possible for you and your child.

CHAPTER 86

Party Time!

Manage and Enjoy Your Autistic Child's Birthday

Tips by Cathy Purple Cherry, AIA, LEED AP

I have experienced sixteen birthdays over our adopted autistic son's nineteen-year life and twenty-five combined birthday parties for our other two younger typically-developing children during our ASD son's sixteen years. There are several tips to implement to make the birthday parties of your autistic child and his or her siblings' parties more successful. Remember that "managing" and "enjoying" a party are two different expectations and sometimes enjoying a party is not realistic at all but managing a party successfully can be accomplished.

956. When choosing to go out to a restaurant to celebrate, always select a child-friendly restaurant with a noise level of at least 8 out of ten (even if your ASD child is a teenager). Also, always request a table larger than you need. If you do not want to explain why, simply advise you may possibly be expecting more people. Place your autistic child in an area with a lot of room. We learned to never place our son next to or across from his younger siblings as this always led to conflict at the table. On your way to the restaurant, figure out what your ASD child wants to eat so that this frustrating conversation does not occur once seated at the table.

957. Make a clear rule for your ASD child that when celebrating his sibling's birthday, the ASD child cannot select his own outfit to wear. It must be appropriate during this one event of the year. This makes a more successful party for the other children because they are not embarrassed. Our son loves to dress in 1960's disco attire and the outfits can be wild. It was a clear rule that he could never dress this way during his siblings' parties or events at their schools.

Bonus Tip! Do not leave wrapped presents out the day or days before the party as the ASD child may open them early from curiosity, and their impulse may be so strong that they cannot stop. While this may be fine for his own presents, it is not acceptable when these presents belong to one of the siblings. This actually happened in our family during one Christmas year. It was a disaster.

958. For celebrations, lower your expectations of appropriate behavior from your ASD child. Just as with typically-developing children, he is very excited at this time and may have difficulty controlling behaviors.

959. Do not use candles with fire and flames if your ASD child has shown an obsession with fire in the past. This tip also applies to your cooking appliance selection. We do not have gas in our house.

960. Keep the celebration simple. Break it into several days if necessary to include various family members yet reduce the number celebrating at one time. Reducing the activity level will reduce the potential for meltdowns by your ASD child.

961. Throughout the year, have your ASD child provide you with specific things desired for birthday and Christmas presents. Predictability is a good thing and helps support better behaviors.

Worst Case! If birthday celebrations of the past have been nightmares, don't have any more or shift them to times of the day, week, month or year that work best to reduce stress. The actual date is not always clearly understood by the ASD child. Do not feel guilty about needing to change the calendar. As parents, we have told stories for years about the Easter bunny and Santa Claus. As parents, we must make up new stories if necessary to help support greater peace in our home.

962. As your son gets older, find out what he sees as the kind of birthday party he would like. Often we plan parties that we think would be fun, that kids without autism enjoy. However, many children with sensory processing challenges do not enjoy the hustle and bustle and noise of lots of people around, or the possibility of balloons popping. Some kids prefer only two to three people at a time and doing an activity they like. I suggest in this case a few mini parties for your son with his favorite people—a couple at a time. If you want a big party for the family, make it for you, but don't expect your son to want to stay in the room. After all, isn't it about him?

—Chantal Sicile-Kira, www.chantalsicile-kira.com

CHAPTER 87

Gift Ideas

Toys for Autistic Children
Tips by Cathy Purple Cherry, AIA, LEED AP

963. Legos can be great toys for kids with autism if they like to put together and take apart stuff. You will learn this early if you start noticing they are breaking a lot of stuff because of their curiosity to see what things look like inside or how they operate.

964. Make sure that whatever toy you give or buy can be broken without regret as many toys will get broken in your child's life. This is not an intentional action—simply the result of a very curious child wanting to understand better how the toy is made with strong impulses to dismantle anything to see how it works.

965. Toys with compartments, keys, and combinations can really intrigue the autistic child. They enjoy repeating the actions of opening and closing and locking and unlocking over and over.

966. If you do not want to support your autistic child's playing with toy guns, then do not support their making them from other objects like cardboard, toilet paper rolls, or Legos. We found that anything our child obsessed about we worked to constantly remove so as to not feed the obsession. With toy guns, we knew he did not have the judgment to understand the difference between toy and real guns. Thus, ALL guns were off limits.

967. Often, simple, everyday items present successfully as toys. Empty boxes and a roll of tape are simple and safe and work great to provide hours of activity. Dangling keys making interesting noises can be intriguing to some ASD children though for others they will try and place them in any holes and cause possible damage. Old wallets provide hidden compartments for folded paper and collected treasures found from the ground. One of my son's favorite things is duct tape as he makes numerous objects or transforms old things into new play shapes. The behavior of repeating actions was very satisfying to him. Thus taping and re-taping and re-taping provided him with hours of interest.

968. Though this may already be obvious, textured toys can provide great tactile stimulation and squishy toys can provide stress reduction. But, if you don't want the liquid of a squishy toy all over your house, don't give them one filled with liquid. They WILL figure out a way to get it out. The same goes for the textured toys. Picking may be something your child likes to do so do not provide a tactile toy with a well-raised texture as these elements will be picked off.

969.

Sorting things is, at times, very appealing to autistic children as it allows them to organize their world. Thus, depending upon the age of the child, the toys for this application could be very different. For the younger children, colored blocks would work. For the older child, it may be buttons or coins.

Some things to keep in mind:

- Little parts on toys are not a good thing. They can cause frustration and, more significantly, stimulate the interest to take the toy apart.
- Loud, noisy toys do not work—not just because of their possible annoyance to your ASD child but because they may stimulate activity and behaviors that you are trying to reduce.
- Do not provide toys with any sharp corners or edges at any age because, during tantrums, these objects can become weapons both to the autistic child and towards their siblings or your home.

Bonus Tip! Chewy toys of course take care of that oral fixation, but are also quite durable. They are easy to carry wherever you go. Check out SensoryUniversity.com. Also, ask your OT for suggestions.

The following tips are adapted from "How to Choose Toys for Autistic Children" provided by wikiHow, a wiki building the world's largest, highest quality how-to manual. Please edit this article and find author credits at www.wikihow.com/Choose-Toys-for-Autistic-Children. Content on wikiHow can be shared under a Creative Commons License.

970. Always be considerate of the child's ability level. Less-complicated toys may be better for children who are more severely impacted by autism; simple push-button, open and use toys are best. For those children on the more able end of the spectrum, building, creating, discovering, connecting, etc. toys are generally fine. For some autistic children who demonstrate a clear preference for a single interest, you can give toys that reflect this interest. This will definitely engage them. The only risk here is that they can rely too much on their single interest and not be challenged to try and engage in other areas where they are lacking interest.

—www.wikihow.com/Choose-Toys-for-Autistic-Children

971. Don't overdo the functional play. There are times during which it is fine to let your child simply enjoy a line of toys that is pure fun. The difficulty arises when the child prefers this line to all else, so monitor any addictive preferences carefully.

—www.wikihow.com/Choose-Toys-for-Autistic-Children

972. Select quality over quantity. Too many toys is always too many toys. For autistic children, it can feel overwhelming and crowding. It is better to choose one good-quality toy over many cheaper toys that will create great clutter. If you hit the right choice, that one toy will provide many hours of enjoyment.

—www.wikihow.com/Choose-Toys-for-Autistic-Children

973. Search online. There are numerous stores catering to toys for autistic children, offering advice and good ideas. There are also many, many guides on what toys to get for autistic children. Have a good read to inform yourself, and apply the most appropriate ideas to suit your child. Every child is different, and every form of autism is different, and you know your own child's needs and interests better than anyone else.

—www.wikihow.com/Choose-Toys-for-Autistic-Children

974. Art supplies. We can never have too many sets of watercolor paints, washable paints and markers, or too much glue or construction paper. I also like them because they don't take up much space. "Model Magic" by Crayola Inc. was and is a hit with my child. He has made some great little pots that have had staying power. The clay-like substance (if stored at room temperature) also doesn't crumble or make much of a mess.

—Julie M. Lorenzen, "Shopping Tips for Children with Autism or Asperger's Syndrome," www.autism-blog.net/2007 /11/shopping-tips-for-children-with-autism.html

975. Books. They store away easily. Children with autism seem to really appreciate nonfiction books, but fiction can be great too. For younger children, I'd suggest books from the "Best Me You Can Be" series or from the "Mr. and Miss" series by Roger Hargreaves. The former provides great social tips for youngsters, and the latter is a cute little fictional series that puts an emphasis on emotions. Both series are available through Scholastic Books. Books with flaps and textures are also a good idea for younger kids.

> —Julie M. Lorenzen, "Shopping Tips for Children with Autism or Asperger's Syndrome," www.autism-blog.net/2007 /11/shopping-tips-for-children-with-autism.html

976. Small sensory toys. Balls with nubby textures and vibrating toys that operate by pulling a string, etc. have been played with by both of my boys.

> —Julie M. Lorenzen, "Shopping Tips for Children with Autism or Asperger's Syndrome," www.autism-blog.net/2007 /11/shopping-tips-for-children-with-autism.html

....

The Future: Happy 18th Birthday—
Where Do We Go from Here?

The best thing about the future is that it comes only one day at a time.

—Abraham Lincoln

I am not afraid of tomorrow, for I have seen yesterday and I love today.

—William Allen White

As a parent, autism will force you to look into the abyss. You will learn who you truly are, and what is possible!

CHAPTER 88

Transition Planning

The following tips for parents whose children have been served through IEPs or 504 plans are adapted from Michelle Garcia Winner, "Parenting through to Adulthood," Socialthinking.com

977. Don't wait until the legal age of the school's transition plan to start transitioning your child into increasing responsibility and independence. The kids will not willingly go along with this plan to do more, but set an expectation and reward small (very small) steps toward the accomplishment. Don't overly focus on the sneer on their face or the less-than-complimentary words they may say; pick your battles carefully. Subtly praise any step toward being a more responsible member of the family. Withhold treats (video games, cell phones, books, etc.) if they are not trying to be a reasonable member of the house most of the time. To give in to their stormy ways is to reinforce the cloud hanging over your house.

978. The adult world is unaccommodating—a fact that is hard to face for everyone, but is particularly so when our special education teams have tried to serve our kids by accommodating to their disability (to some extent). Prevent the IEP team and yourself from making decisions that always keep your child comfortable and in control of what he wants to do. As parents of young kids, we work to keep our kids comfortable; now we have to work, literally work, to make sure our kids are learning to be comfortable with the fact that the world frequently does not offer "comfortable" options.

979. Problem-solving is about finding the least painful option, not the one that causes no pain. Problem-solving often does not actually solve the problem! Assure you child, "Yes, you hate the teacher, but you've got to learn to deal with it! You may hate a boss one day!" Parents then need to make sure they don't step in to intervene, to try and solve their children's problems for them. There is a tendency when we identify a child with a disability to make the child's disability everyone else's problem, but by the time they graduate from school, it is totally their challenge to deal with, mostly on their own. While there will be some special people to reach out and continue to help, especially while they are in their young twenties, the "game" has changed significantly. Our kids are expected to do much more for themselves the year after they graduate from high school than the year before. Plan for this ahead of time!

980. Avoid burnout. Something the parents of my clients have taught me over the years is that they wear out! Begin to work on all of the above slowly but surely when your child is thirteen, fourteen, fifteen. They may have been happy to drive their child to high school, but they no longer want to drive their child to college, or their job, nor should they! The social rules have changed, and it is so incredibly unhip to be driven around by your parents when you are a young adult. You won't regret it. Your child won't be ready to fly solo (very likely) by the time they graduate from high school (nor were my daughters!), but they will be more on their way and slowly be able to handle the growing pressures of having to do more for themselves, even if they don't want to.

981. Our children's self-esteem is born from the recognition of their own accomplishments and not on just "being smart" or being told they are wonderful. Show them how to appreciate that feeling good about the fact you can do things in your community for yourself is at least as important (or more important) than getting good grades on tests. The world has a lot of smart people in it; what the adult world really celebrates are people who can figure out how to work as a member of society, which means working reasonably well with other people.

982. Teach your children your own experience, what you know yourself. Your lessons of how to be a more effective adult continue to be learned across your life. Help them to know that the process of learning about being a citizen of the world is not like graduating from high school; there is no diploma, and it never ends. But a growing sense of maturity is something to be proud of.

983. If it's not working . . . All this being said, if you think your child's challenges are far, far larger and his mood far, far darker, before putting any more demands on your child, first go to a psychologist/counselor to seek an assessment and guidance about how to help with possible mental health challenges (e.g., depression and/or anxiety) that may need to be addressed before adding more pressure at a confusing period of development for us all!

984. Some people on the more-able end of the spectrum learn to drive. However, it may take longer to learn because of their sensory processing and motor coordination challenges. The easy part tends to be learning the rules involved in driving.

985. Negative public perceptions and gender stereotypes can present multiple barriers to future planning. Planning for the future requires that all members of the team have high expectations and not limit themselves by stereotypes. Parents and professionals must fight actively against such limiting ideas.

—Lori Ernsperger, PhD and Danielle Wendel,
Girls Under the Umbrella of Autism Spectrum Disorders

CHAPTER 89

Getting a Job

The following tips are from Denise Zangoglia, "8 Top Tips-
Planning For Life After High School For Your Autistic Child,"
EpilepsyMoms.com, www.epilepsymoms.com/disease/autism/8-
top-tips-planning-life-after-high-school-your-autistic-child.html

Make sure your child takes a career assessment test for some initial
direction that can help the student focus on the concrete rather
than the abstract. It's imperative to stay involved and keep on top
of the process even if you think the school is handling it. Look
into options on your own. Some agencies, such as the Department
of Vocational Rehabilitation, Social Security Administration, or
independent and supported living centers, might provide training
or direct services to assist the school with a student's transition.
Local public schools are required by law to supply information
about these services as part of transition planning in high school.

There should be a master plan with short- and long-range goals
and the tasks or activities that are required to achieve those goals.
The goals and services will be dependent on the needs, skills, and
personal preferences of each child. Parents can help their son or
daughter by assigning some chores or arranging for volunteer
work to discover whether or not they want a structured work
environment or a competitive job. The options to consider for
post high school life are:

- Vocational training
- Community interaction and participation

- Level of independent living skills
- Adult services offered
- Postsecondary education
- Adult and continuing education
- Integrated and/or supported employment

Consider your child's strengths and interests and don't discount splinter skills (strengths that might be out of proportion to their other skills). Focus on those, as they can be the foundation for thriving in continuing education, employment, and socialization. This can range from careers as musicians, mathematicians, artists, structural designers with mechanical or spatial skills; mathematical calculation skills, athletic performance; and computer ability.

986. Ask career/vocational questions. It's important that the parents, the child, the teachers, siblings, and other significant persons in your child's life be a part of this, as each can offer valuable insights. Some questions to start the ball rolling are listed below, and in the course of asking them, other questions that are pertinent will come up. Add to and refine your list as you go through the process to develop the best direction for your child.

- What does your son/daughter like to do?
- What can they do?
- What needs to be explored more?
- What skills or information does your son/daughter need to learn and understand to reach their goals?
- How does college fit in the picture for them? Four-year, community, vocational, or adult education?

- What options/services are available for learning about employment and/or training?
- Where will your son/daughter live?
- How does a job sound to your child, either supportive or competitive?
- How will they support themselves?
- How will they acquire health insurance?
- Will your child require help and support from you? (You might want to see an attorney who deals specifically with special-needs trusts, if this is the case)
- What kind of transportation is available for your child?

987. Ask social interactive questions. Life after high school must also take into account the social network of your child. Friends, community, and a sense of belonging are just as important factors.

- Does your child have the skills to form and foster friendships, or will they need help and encouragement?
- Is your child known in the community through volunteer, sports, creative arts, or religious affiliations?
- Does your son or daughter have a hobby or passion? Are they involved in a horseback-riding program, music program, or club that others might share an interest in as an activity?
- What venues are available for socializing? For example: choir, sports/team recordkeeping/statistician, religious affiliations, senior center involvement, fire department volunteer helper.

988. Take action. As with anything, planning is not enough. Follow-through is key to a successful venture. If your child is especially gifted with math or computer skills, see if you can arrange to acquire a position for them in a data services job. They will learn the office and social skills and procedures appropriate for a work environment. This might involve clocking in or following a scheduled work task list, or even giving them the right amount of time to get to work on time. Making sure your child can sit for certain length of time required in a work environment is crucial.

989. Try to offer them the tools to help them decide if this environment is one they might want to explore. You might also consider setting up a section of your home or home office for them as a practice work environment. My sister-in-law did this for her child to acclimate him to a simulated work environment. She furnished it with the necessary technology, as well as furnishings such as a desk, ergonomic mesh chair, and photos of the things he loved to make him feel comfortable.

990. Many businesses offer employment in different capacities, such as packaging companies that require assembly with a requirement for accuracy and a deadline, and uniform service companies that require sorting and cleaning. U.S. military installations are very supportive by offering positions that involve copying, folding, sealing, and mailing newsletters. The skills needed and required are neatness and completion of tasks in a timely manner.

991. For outdoor or non-office work, consider jobs such as community cleanup, store greeter, restaurant host/hostess, a cleaning job, industrial arts, home maintenance, mobile work crew opportunities such as lawn care and maintenance, and janitorial services. By offering a student the opportunity to experience numerous and diverse work settings and acquire the necessary and suitable skills, the child will be more comfortable with the decision and be able to choose the best path.

992. The mind-set of parents: This is a tough one, as it is so hard to push a child we feel/know might have a more difficult time than others, but you might be doing them a disservice. What we thought as limiting possibilities might be shattered, and your child might exceed your expectations and limited beliefs. To read more on this topic of possibility thinking, go to http://GoldenMailbox.com/library and http://GoldenMailbox.com/newsletters.

993. Know the contacts: To prepare your child, know who to contact for help. Employment-related service agencies might not get involved until your child is close to graduating from high school. Do a search online for services in your state. In New Jersey within the Department of Labor there is the Division of Vocational Rehabilitation Services (DVRS). They help people with disabilities to prepare for, obtain, and keep a job. They offer services such as:

- Diagnostic Services
- Vocational Evaluation
- Counseling
- Placement
- Follow-up services
- Post-employment services
- Physical restoration
- Job coaching; vocational, professional or on-the-job training

994. Some job tips for people with autism or Asperger's syndrome:
- Jobs should have a well-defined goal or endpoint.
- Sell your work, not your personality. Make a portfolio of your work.
- The boss must recognize your social limitations.
  —Temple Grandin, PhD, author of *Thinking in Pictures* and *The Way I See It*; www.autism.com/ind_choosing_job.asp

995. It is important that high-functioning autistics and Asperger's syndrome people pick a college major in an area where they can get jobs. Computer science is a good choice because it is very likely that many of the best programmers have either Asperger's syndrome or some of its traits. Other good majors are: accounting, engineering, library science, and art, with an emphasis on commercial art and drafting. Majors in history, political science, business, English, or pure math should be avoided. However, one could major in library science with a minor in history, but the library science degree makes it easier to get a good job.
  —Temple Grandin, PhD, author of *Thinking in Pictures* and *The Way I See It*; www.autism.com/ind_choosing_job.asp

996. Some individuals, while they are still in high school, should be encouraged to take courses at a local college in drafting, computer programming, or commercial art. This will help keep them motivated and serve as a refuge from teasing. Families with low incomes may be wondering how they can afford computers for their child to learn programming or computer-aided drafting. Used computers can often be obtained for free or at a very low cost when a business or an engineering company upgrades their equipment. Many people do not realize that there are many usable older computers sitting in storerooms at schools, banks, factories, and other businesses. It will not be the latest new thing, but it is more than adequate for a student to learn on.

—Temple Grandin, PhD, author of *Thinking in Pictures* and *The Way I See It*; www.autism.com/ind_choosing_job.asp

CHAPTER 90

Attending College

997. If your teenage son is headed for college, he will need to get prepared for this change in physical and social environment. Plan a trip to the college and show him where the library, the bookstore, the cafeteria, health services, and so on are located. Then, you can explain how to handle everyday situations that could come up in college, such as "Where do I go to buy personal care products if I run out?" or "What do I do if I missed a class because I woke up late?"

The following tips are provided by Lars Perner, PhD (www.AspergersSyndrome.org).

Choosing a College

- It is tempting to consider getting a start at a community college (CC) rather than at a university, and there are situations where this may be useful.
- Temple Grandin—a hero to many of us!—has very insightfully recommended that high school students with special interests and/or greater advancement in certain subjects take courses at a CC during the school year and/or over the summer. If the student is already familiar with the CC that way, the transition may be smoother. . . . A CC may also be located more conveniently, allowing the student to live at home, or at least closer to home.
- The quality of instruction at both CCs and four-year colleges varies widely, so it is difficult to say whether substantive learning will suffer. Students will probably get more individual attention at a community

---

college than they would at a research oriented university where many of the freshperson and sophomore courses are taught in the infamous four hundred student lecture halls.

- One option is to consider a technical program, or trade school, rather than a traditional university education. Here, the student will have the opportunity to focus more explicitly on his or her interests.

- Many private colleges provide significantly smaller classes and more individual attention. However, the price tag can be quite prohibitive.

- A number of public teaching oriented universities may provide a good solution. I was fortunate to go to the Cal Poly, which provided an excellent quality of education. A guidance counselor may be able to offer some good advice on available options within an acceptable distance from home.

Securing Needed Services

- Individuals with autism vary tremendously in the help and services they will need to function effectively, and colleges differ a great deal in what they offer.

- The issue arises as to how much a student should disclose to his or her professors, and what, if any, accommodations he or she should request. This is an individual matter, and the answer will vary depending on the individual case and the student's relative desire for privacy. Theoretically, in the United States, the Americans with Disabilities Act requires educational institutions and employers to provide the disabled with "reasonable accommodations." In practice, however, the act has been described as lacking "teeth" and exactly what it mandates is not at all clear. Many universities explicitly require that any special accommodations must be requested through the disabled student services office rather than directly to a professor. The type of campus involved is likely to make a significant difference. Faculty in small liberal arts colleges are likely to be a lot more accommodating than those in big research institutions, where teaching and individuals are more likely to be seen as obstacles to research.

- Most colleges offer some counseling services, which are often quite in demand among a large proportion of students struggling to adjust to various phases of college life. These counseling services may or may not have staff experienced in dealing with students on the spectrum and even when they do, students may be eligible for only a small number of sessions. University health centers vary somewhat in what kinds of required medial services they may offer.

Moving Away to College and Pragmatics

- For some students on the spectrum, academics are the easy stuff, and the real trouble involves moving away from home and coping with the pragmatics of independent and group living.

- For those going to a college "far away" (a term that will have different meanings to different people), one of the problems is that the transition is so abrupt. You leave one day, arriving perhaps a week before the start of the term. And many of the other pressures are likely to start at the same time.

- If a student is within driving distance, feels comfortable driving, and has a car, he or she can have the assurance of being able to come home—if he or she feels the urge to do so—every week-end if need be. The beauty of a safety net is that its existence does not mean that it actually has to be used—but it can go a long way in quelling anxiety. . . . For those who live farther away from home, open-ended bus, train, or plane tickets or vouchers, for those who can afford them, can provide a real sense of security.

- One very important issue is living arrangements. It is easy to visualize how disastrous a residence hall can be to an individual with autism. Having to share a room with someone else (a reality in most residence halls), lack of privacy in bathrooms, and the crowded and noisy quarters sound quite hellish, and I am glad I never had to go through that experience. Cafeteria food may or may not be a problem. At least there is frequently a lot of choice, and you don't have to prepare the food yourself.

Chapter 91

Special-Needs Trusts

998. A special-needs trust (SNT) serves two primary functions: First, it provides management of funds for your son should he not be able to do so himself, and second, it preserves your son's eligibility for public benefits, including Medicaid, SSI, or any other program.

- The SNT allows you to leave resources for his benefit without cutting off public assistance (Medicaid and such) and ensures that your other children will not be overburdened with his care.
- The SNT will make sure that any funds left to your son will be properly managed and distributed, and it provides fair allocation between your kids.
- You may think you do not need a SNT currently, but remember that things change; public programs change over the years, and siblings may have their own difficulties. A SNT can provide a secure future for your son.
- To create the SNT you will need the help of a lawyer with experience in SNTs. Ask other parents for references; contact your Medicaid coordinator, as these organizations sometimes provide discounted or free legal help. Ask your current lawyers covering other areas of your life for a referral.
- Together with your legal and financial advisors, you will choose an appropriate trustee who will manage the SNT.
- When meeting with the above professionals, assess your current situation, analyze the impact of the plan on your estate and aid programs, and then adjust as necessary.

....

Finances—Supporting the War Effort

A small leak will sink a great ship.

                                    —*Benjamin Franklin as Poor Richard*

For age and want save while you may,
No morning sun lasts a whole day.

                                    —*Benjamin Franklin as Poor Richard*

CHAPTER 92

Tax Season—Christmas in April?

999. While reviewing your taxes, should you notice a benefit that you missed claiming in past years, you may file an amended return within three years of the date that you filed the original return.

1000. Additional caregivers, such as grandparents, aunts and uncles, and even nonrelatives caretakers, may qualify for tax benefits through various means. Be sure to mention any funds used to help the child (even if not your own) to your tax preparer. Please make sure you meet the requirements, though, as this is pretty tightly regulated by the IRS.

1001. Ask your son's various physicians, therapists, and other professionals for a letter stating what treatments, therapies, and or meds they require on an annual basis and file it. Should the IRS audit you regarding medical expense deductions, these letters will prove invaluable.

Tax Tips by Kim Mack Rosenberg
and Mark L. Berger, CPA

The information contained herein is for informational purposes only and does not substitute for tax advice from your own tax adviser, familiar with your financial information. While they have endeavored to be as accurate as possible, the authors make no warranties, express or implied, concerning the information contained herein. As always, official sources and publications and your own tax professional should be consulted for the most current rules and regulations that may be applicable to you.

- Medical expenses above the first 7.5 percent of your adjusted gross income are tax-deductible. Medical expenses up to the first 7.5 percent of adjusted gross income are never deductible (even when your expenses exceed 7.5 percent of your adjusted gross income; only the excess is deductible).
- Save medical receipts for your entire family, even if you don't think you will qualify for a medical expense deduction. You never know when a catastrophic medical bill or a change in family finances could happen and put you over the 7.5 percent threshold.

- IRS publication 502, available at www.IRS.gov, is a great resource to determine what is deductible. Pub. 502 also lists expenses that generally are not deductible, but exceptions in those categories often allow deductions for some of the medical care required by special-needs children.

- Get a letter from a doctor(s) substantiating your child's need for his treatments and related expenses, like occupational therapy, physical therapy, speech therapy, supplements, special toys/equipment, homeopathy, hyperbaric treatment, the need for you to attend conferences/buy books related to your child's condition or treatment, typical classes (for socialization, for example, if essential to your child's treatment). If you make this an easy step for your practitioners, they are usually amenable to helping you—they want your child to get the treatments he or she needs, too! Keep this letter in case of audit.

- Supplements that are recommended by a medical practitioner to treat a medical condition diagnosed by a doctor may be deductible, but supplements taken for general "good health" reasons are not deductible.

- Tuition for a therapeutic school generally will qualify as a medical expense, but if you are reimbursed for that tuition in a later tax year, you will have to account for the reimbursement, and, under some circumstances, some portion could count as income. Reimbursements (including insurance reimbursements) are taxable to the extent that the expense was deducted. If you don't deduct the tuition and then don't get reimbursed, you have three

- years from the date that you filed that year's return to go back and amend your return.
- For car travel for medical purposes, you can deduct the larger of the statutory mileage rate (it changes each year and is different for medical vs. business) or your actual expenses (gas and oil, primarily). Tolls and parking are deductible in addition to either actual costs or the statutory per mile deduction. If you use your car in connection with medical expenses and take the standard medical mileage rate deduction, you should keep a mileage log (you can even keep it in the car to be sure to have it when you need it).
- Conferences fees and transportation expenses for conferences you attend to learn about your child's medical condition/treatment are includable medical expenses; however, meals and lodging at the conference are not.
- The cost of travel (including an accompanying parent's costs) to another city for medical care is deductible if the primary purpose of your trip is to treat a medical condition. Lodging (at a statutorily defined rate) also is deductible when traveling out of town for medical treatment.
- However, meals are not deductible (except for the patient in a hospital or similar facility).
- The *difference* between the cost of foods for special diets (such as the gluten-free/casein-free diet) versus "normal" equivalents is deductible when the special diet is prescribed by a doctor to alleviate a medical condition. For a handy template on these sometimes-complicated calculations, check out www.TACAnow.org.

- You should evaluate employer-provided plans such as a flex spending plan, because it gives you the opportunity to pay for medical expenses with pre-tax earnings.

- Medical expenses reimbursed by a flex spending plan do not qualify as medical expenses for tax deduction purposes—you paid for this with pre-tax dollars and cannot "double dip." (In other words, if you were reimbursed by flex spending, you cannot claim the expense on your taxes).

- Insurance premiums paid with pre-tax dollars (which is the case for many employees) are *not* deductible. If you are self-employed, these premiums may be subject to different tax treatment (not as a medical expense).

- In balancing flex-spending dollars vs. insurance coverage, if you think an expense may be covered by your insurance, submit it to your insurer first. Use your flex spending dollars wisely.

- Expenses not covered by insurance and not tax deductible may still be eligible for flex spending. These items even include some OTC medications. Consult your flex spending account information on reimbursable items. If you can use pre-tax dollars to be repaid for items that are not tax-deductible, it might make sense to use flex-spending dollars for those items before potentially tax-deductible items.

- Payments for medical expenses necessary to meet your insurance policy deductible as well as co-pays after you meet your deductible are tax-deductible.

- The best practice is to keep receipts and to document everything in case of an audit.

- Documentation of medical expenses should include the

name and address of the person you paid and the amount
and date you paid, a description of the service/goods
provided, and the date provided.

- Try not to pay medical expenses with cash—credit cards
  and checks are easier to substantiate.

- If your child/family has a lot of medical expenses, stay
  on top of filing regularly. If your paperwork builds up,
  items may go missing and the task becomes too daunting.
  Create a filing system that works for you.

- Submit each claim to your insurer separately, one claim
  per envelope. Claims are less likely to be lost if they arrive
  separately rather than in bulk.

- Keep a copy of the claim form and provider's bill/
  receipt in case the insurer misplaces the claim and you
  need to resubmit, and to help you keep track of paid and
  outstanding claims. Note the date you sent it on your
  copy. When you receive an explanation of benefits from
  your insurer, you can attach it to these documents.

- Learn how to read your insurer's "explanation of benefits"
  to determine what is tax-deductible on a given claim and
  to be sure you are accounting for all potential deductions.
  Any deduction is based on what remains after the charge
  is reduced based on any agreement your doctor or other
  provider may have with the insurer, and after your insurer
  pays its share. These may include: "not covered amounts";
  co-pays; deductibles; and co-insurance (for example, if
  you have a 70/30 plan—your 30 percent share of the
  allowed charge is a deductible medical expense).

- To help you and your tax preparer prepare your return
  efficiently and accurately, create a document (in a word
  processing, database, or spreadsheet program with which

you are comfortable), or use a money management program that allows you to track the expenses by category or groups of categories. If you create a document, you can use the same document and save it as a new version each year—no need to reinvent the wheel.

Conclusion

....

I just threw 1,001 tips at you. How do you feel? I know there is a lot to consider and sample. Just try and keep things as simple as possible when looking at these tips. View the process as iterative: Some will work for you, and some will not. Take those that work for you and gradually work them into your daily routine.

It is my hope that you will discover even one tip in this compilation that will have a positive impact on your child's life, and your own. Write and tell us about it. We'd also love to hear any tips you may have. Send them to us, and they could make the next edition and land you a free copy of the book. E-mail us at autism@skyhorsepublishing.com.

I cannot resist one last quote:

> Remember, Red—hope is a good thing, maybe the best of things.
> —*Andy Dufresne (played by Tim Robbins),*
> The Shawshank Redemption

PS: Look for us on the *Psychology Today* blog at www.psychologytoday.com /blog/dads-diary.

Acknowledgments

....

I am deeply indebted to in-house Skyhorse Publishing editor Joseph Sverchek, without whom I could not possibly have completed this project. I would also like to thank Chantal Sicile-Kira (internationally recognized autism author, advocate, and speaker), Jane Johnson (Managing Director of the Autism Research Institute), Kim Mack-Rosenberg (Vice President National Autism Association, New York Metro Chapter), Cathy Purple Cherry (AIA, LEED-AP, Principal of Purple Cherry Architects), and Teri Arranga (Director of AutismOne) for all their comments and suggestions; they helped bring this project to another level.

And special thanks go to the hundreds of parents, writers, teachers, therapists, doctors, and others whose thoughts, ideas, and words of wisdom are contained in this book.

Suggested Reading

....

Books

7 Kinds of Smart (Plume, 1999) by Thomas Armstrong.

41 Things to Know About Autism (Turner, 2010) by Chantal Sicile-Kira.

1001 Great Ideas for Teaching and Raising Children with Autism Spectrum Disorders (Future Horizons, 2010) by Ellen Notbohm and Veronica Zysk.

Adolescents on the Autism Spectrum: A Parent's Guide to the Cognitive, Social, Physical, and Transition Needs of Teenagers with Autism Spectrum Disorders (Penguin, 2006) by Chantal Sicile-Kira. Foreword by Temple Grandin, PhD. 2006 San Diego Book Award for "Best in Health/Fitness."

All I Can Handle: I'm No Mother Theresa (Skyhorse, 2010) by Kim Stagliano.

Autism: A Holistic Approach (Floris Books, 2002) by Bob Woodward and Dr. Marga Hogenboom.

Autism Life Skills: From Communication and Safety to Self Esteem and More: 10 Essential Abilities Every Child Deserves and Needs to Learn (Penguin, 2008) by Chantal Sicile-Kira. Foreword by Temple Grandin, PhD.

Autism Spectrum Disorders: The Complete Guide to Understanding Autism, Asperger's Syndrome, Pervasive Developmental Disorder, and other ASD's (Penguin, 2005) by Chantal Sicile-Kira, Foreword by Temple Grandin, PhD. Recipient of 2005 Autism Society of America's Outstanding Literary Work of the Year Award. Nominated for the 2005 PEN/Martha Albrand Award for First Nonfiction.

Autistic Spectrum Disorders: Understanding the Diagnosis and Getting Help (O'Reilly & Associates, 2002) by Mitzi Waltz.

Changing the Course of Autism (Sentient, 2007) by Bryan Jepson, MD with Jane Johnson.

Children and Youth with Asperger's Syndrome (Corwin, 2005) by Brenda Smith-Myles.

Children with Starving Brains (Bramble, 2009) by Jaquelyn McCandless.

Cutting-Edge Therapies for Autism 2010–2011 (Skyhorse, 2010) by Ken Siri and Tony Lyons

Engaging Autism (Da Capo, 2009) by Stanley Greenspan, MD.

Getting Beyond Bullying and Exclusion PreK–5 (Corwin, 2009) by Ronald Mah.

Girls Under the Umbrella of Autism Spectrum Disorders (Autism Asperger Press, 2007) by Lori Ernsperger, PhD, and Danielle Wendel.

Healing our Autistic Children (Palgrave Macmillan, 2010) by Julie A. Buckley, MD.

Healing the New Childhood Epidemics (Ballantine, 2008) by Kenneth Bock, MD.

Helping Children with Autism Learn (Oxford, 2007) by Bryna Siegel.

Other Neurological Differences (Autism Asperger Publishing, 2005) by Lisa Lieberman.

Overcoming ADHD (Da Capo, 2009) by Stanley Greenspan, MD.

Physicians' Desk Reference (PDR Network, 2009) by PDR Staff.

Poor Richards Almanac (Random House, 1988) by Benjamin Franklin.

Son-Rise: The Miracle Continues (HJ Kramer, 1995) by Barry Neil Kaufman and Raun Kaufman.

Stumbling on Happiness (Vintage, 2007) by Daniel Gilbert

Teaching Students with Autism Spectrum Disorders (Corwin, 2008) by Roger Pierangelo and George A. Giuliani.

Suggested Reading

The Art of War (Shambhala, 2005), by Sun Tzu, translation Thomas Cleary.

The Autism Book (Little, Brown, 2010) by Robert Sears, MD.

The Autism Sourcebook (Harper, 2006) by Karen Siff Exkorn.

The Complete IEP Guide: How to Advocate for Your Special Ed Child (NOLO. 2009) by Lawrence Siegel.

The Encyclopedia of Dietary Interventions for the Treatment of Autism and Related Disorders (Sarpsborg Press, 2008) by Karyn Seroussi and Lisa Lewis, PhD.

The Everyday Advocate (NAL, 2010) by Areva Martin, Esq. and Lynn Kern Koegel.

The Hidden Curriculum: Practical Solutions for Understanding Unstated Rules in Social Solutions (Autism Asperger Publishing, 2004) by Brenda Smith-Myles.

The Mindbody Prescription (Warner, 1999) by John Sarno, M.D.

The Way I See It (Future Horizons, 2008) by Temple Grandin, PhD.

The Way They Learn (Tyndale House, 1998) by Cynthia Ulrich Tobias

Thinking in Pictures (Vintage, 2010) by Temple Grandin, PhD.

Three Times the Love (Avery, 2009) by Lynn and Randy Gaston.

We Band of Mothers (Autism Research Institute, 2007) by Judy Chinitz.

What Your Doctor May Not Tell You About(TM) Children's Vaccinations (Grand Central, 2007) by Stephanie Cave, MD.

Magazines

ARRI Quarterly
Spectrum Magazine
The Advocate
The Autism File